Men and Maternity

Since the development of modern medicine men have become increasingly involved in childbearing as obstetricians and, more recently, as fathers. Childbearing has been revolutionised due, in no small part, to the involvement of men.

This book argues that the beneficial contribution of men has been taken for granted. Certain changes to childbearing practice have resulted, which, together with men's involvement, have been encouraged without any reference to evidence and without adequate opportunity for reflection.

Considering the findings of recent research and wider literature, and using qualitative research with mothers, *Men and Maternity*

- traces the beginning of men's involvement in childbearing in practising interventive medicine
- discusses the medicalisation of childbirth and highlights the potential for iatrogenesis for the mother and child due to unnecessary interventions
- looks at the difficulties men experience with childbirth as fathers and their responses to these difficulties
- gives attention to certain particularly challenging situations, such as fathers' grief
- analyses the taken-for-granted assumptions about the beneficial contribution men make to childbearing, both as practitioners and as fathers, and asks whether there may also be disadvantages.

This book is the first to question assumptions about the beneficial involvement of men in childbearing. It will therefore be of great interest to academics and postgraduate students of midwifery, obstetrics, medicine and health studies, as well as practising midwives and obstetricians, health visitors, childbirth educators and labour and delivery room nurses.

Rosemary Mander is Reader in Nursing Studies at the University of Edinburgh. She has almost forty years' experience of midwifery practice, working alongside men and with men as fathers. She has published widely on childbearing and midwifery.

Men and Maternity

Rosemary Mander

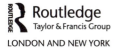
Routledge
Taylor & Francis Group

LONDON AND NEW YORK

First published 2004
by Routledge
11 New Fetter Lane, London EC4P 4EE

Simultaneously published in the USA and Canada
by Routledge
29 West 35th Street, New York, NY 10001

Routledge is an imprint of the Taylor & Francis Group

© 2004 Rosemary Mander

Typeset in Sabon by
Keystroke, Jacaranda Lodge, Wolverhampton
Printed and bound in Great Britain by
TJ International Ltd, Padstow, Cornwall

British Library Cataloguing in Publication Data
A catalogue record for this book is available from the British Library

Library of Congress Cataloging in Publication Data
A catalog record for this book has been requested

ISBN 0–415–27580–6 (hbk)
ISBN 0–415–27587–3 (pbk)

Contents

Acknowledgements

I would like to acknowledge the help of a number of people who have unstintingly shared their time and their ideas. Obviously, though, the thoughts in this book derive from these people's ideas being reframed by me, which means that the material is my responsibility.

I am grateful to Dr Martin P. Johnson, Dr Elizabeth R. Perkins, Tandy Deane-Gray and the RCM Library for helping me with access to material. I appreciate the work of Chris Bewley in reading Chapter 6 and Professor Kerry Jacobs for reading Chapter 5. Also appreciated is the contribution of Dr Lindsay Reid for her interest and enthusiasm. My thanks go to Lynn Kilbride and Mike Ramsay for their recollections. The help of Jenny Gould in the preparation of the manuscript is appreciated.

I would like to express my gratitude to Lindsay Sedgeworth for persuading me, perhaps inadvertently, that this book is necessary.

I would also like to recognise the input of all the men I have ever had the joy of working with.

My sincere thanks go to the women I interviewed for the research mentioned in Chapter 7 and the Iolanthe Trust who funded this work.

Most of all my infinite gratitude goes to Iain Abbot, who is the exception that really does prove the rule.

Introduction

The menfolk

The childbearing scenario is the unequivocal focus of this book. As with any great story, the major focal point is likely to be found in the *dramatis personae*, rather than in the plot as such. The main actor, of course, is the woman in the process of becoming a mother. She has traditionally and rightly been the major focus of attention for all those involved in childbearing.

It may be, though, that her role as *prima donna* is under threat of being usurped by a range of techniques, interventions and bit players. Two of the relatively recent arrivals on the childbearing scene, the baby's father and the medical practitioner, appear to be particularly guilty of threatening to steal the woman's limelight. In view of this, the purpose of this book is to examine the nature of these men's input into the childbearing scenario. In doing this I will assess the existence, reality and extent of any threat which they may present.

Who the man is

Throughout this book I attempt, as far as possible, to refer to the man in the singular. This is because the generalisation, which a plural would imply, may not be appropriate for such a varied constituency. Having clarified that the focus is on the individuals, it is necessary to explain that those individuals belong to one of two groups, although some may belong to both. These two groups of men are the partners and the attendants; that is, the medical personnel. Although the term 'partner' is less than ideal, it is widely understood and probably accurate, whereas 'husband' in Western Europe is becoming increasingly likely to be imprecise.

At first glance, it may appear that the father and the medical practitioner have very little in common. On the basis of the literature, the assumption is being made throughout this book that their gender, or at least their gender attributes, are widely shared (see Chapter 2, pp. 36–7), although some may question this. Other, more specific commonalities will manifest themselves as the book progresses.

Who the man is not

There are two other groups of males to whom I will not specifically be giving attention.

The boy baby

Being a boy baby may be said to be a mixed blessing. While more boys are conceived and born than are girl babies, they tend to be less healthy. Thus the female/male ratio is approximately equal by the time adulthood is reached (Lorber, 1997: 18). It has recently been suggested that, even as a fetus, the boy may make greater demands than his sister on his mother's resources. This is through an association with an increased dietary energy intake in the pregnant woman who is carrying a boy baby (Tamimi *et al.*, 2003).

The grandfather

Unlike the grandmother who is an ongoing source of assistance, support and consolation, the grandfather tends not to feature in the childbearing scenario. The exception is the grandfather of the baby being relinquished for adoption (See Chapter 7), where the situation is very different. A survey with some qualitative elements (Wenger and Burholt, 2001) found that relations with the grandfather became less intense as the young person became an adult. Perhaps not surprisingly, the factor which was the strongest influence on the maintenance of contact was the existence of capital, or some other form of property, which could be available to be inherited. This may be another example of the relatively short-term influence of the man.

The context

There are a small number of situational aspects which have influenced the development of the ideas in this book. These aspects are both different and differently significant. In addition, they apply unequally to the two main groups of men.

Power relationships

> One concept which needs to be taken into account from the outset is one of which the men in the childbearing scenario, and possibly some women, may not be aware. Other women may deny that it is any longer a problem – if it has ever existed. The concept which needs to be borne in mind is patriarchal power, which is defined as: Systemic societal structures that institutionalise male physical, social and economic power over women.
>
> (Reeves and Baden, 2000)

Although the concept of patriarchy may be helpful to some women to the point of being liberating, this is not universally the case (Bryson, 1999). The concept of patriarchy has been condemned by some feminist critics on the grounds that it is part of the problem rather than the solution. Patriarchy has been labelled as a construct created by members of the white middle classes to shore up their own position of strength. Equally, it has been criticised for being too trite. In this way it may be seen as limiting debate and stifling discussion by effectively putting the lid on the difficult questions, rather than opening them up to interrogation, analysis and debate.

The term 'patriarchy' as a form of misuse of power was first introduced to the feminist literature by Kate Millett in 1971. To develop this persuasive argument, she applied the anti-Vietnam and civil rights and student rights political activism of the 1960s to the situations in which women found themselves. In this way women were made to realise that their supposedly individual experiences of underachievement, unhappy relationships and domestic violence were far from unique. These experiences were found to be common enough to justify the recognition of a widespread abuse of male hegemony. Perhaps unfortunately, it was from this recognition that the all too familiar epigram was coined: 'The personal is political'.

The universality of male power is, according to Millett, one of the factors which renders it pervasive to the point of invisibility. Unlike other forms of oppression, patriarchy is not confined to any particular century, socio-economic class or ethnic group. Its ubiquity carries with it the menace of the widespread assumption that it is the natural order of things.

The oppression of women has often been shown to feature most frequently in work in the home, in paid employment, in statutory structures, in culture, in sexuality and in criminal violence. Because the roles of men and women are more clearly delineated in reproductive functioning, this may not be regarded as a site of women's oppression. It has been argued, though, that this is far from the case (Mander and Reid, 2002: 14). One of the ways in which this oppression has been identified is found in the writing of Pollack and Sutton (1985). These authors are unwilling to interpret the father's increasing involvement in childbearing as the saccharine experience to which it is often compared. Instead, they reinterpret his involvement as another example of men exerting their rights at the expense of their women partners.

In this book I advance the argument that the men who are intended to provide care for the childbearing woman are, each for his own individual reasons, unable to do so. While they certainly do not intend to cause her harm, they find themselves in unforeseen situations in which they are unable to behave in anything other than predetermined ways. The result, for a number of reasons which will become apparent below, is a deterioration in the woman's experience of childbearing. This result may further involve a range of phenomena which, ultimately, cause iatrogenic effects for her baby, as well as for the woman herself.

New fathering in the media

The other main contextual aspect which has influenced the development of this book is, arguably, a more recent phenomenon. This is the man who claims or is described as being a 'new father' or a 'nurturant father' (Storr, 2003: 41). Probably originating in North America, this idea is another by-product of the counterculture of the 1960s. Lamb (1986), however, maintains that this man came into being as late as the mid-1970s.

The new father has been given a good press. To the extent that he exists, he has enjoyed the wealth of publicity which has focused solely on the benefits of men's input into childbearing. The media appear to relish the story which they have cornered on doting and dutiful dads. These journalistic embellishments appear to provide the perfect complement to their other birth story stock in trade – that of the medical miracle. The reality of the father's contribution will become apparent as this book scrutinises the research literature on the birth process. The rhetoric, however, is well exemplified in the website of the National Childbirth Trust (1998). This website includes two pages entitled 'Becoming a Dad'. One page is headed 'Your role at the birth' and the other 'Practical steps to help your partner'.

A selection of fathers' comments are provided. They include the following:

> 'This was a wonderful experience and one that I am glad that I did not miss.'
> 'I would have been nowhere else that evening.'
> 'I was able to help Sarah to cope with the contractions by massaging her back and suggesting new positions.'
> 'One thing I felt able to help with was to help Judie use gas and air during contractions. I feel competent with machines, so this felt like something I could contribute.'

Of the nine quotations in this section of the website, eight are similar to the four quoted above. The other quotation shows somewhat less unalloyed delight:

> 'For many men witnessing the birth of their child is a fantastic, life-enhancing experience. Others don't give it such rave reviews.'

The latter seven words are the only indication on the website that there may be a less than totally positive side to this experience.

The old adage 'Don't let the truth spoil a good story' is clearly the agenda here. While there is no suggestion that these are anything other than genuine comments, this book will show that such a positive bias in no way echoes the experience of a large number of men as reflected in the research findings. This misrepresentation of the father's reality may be seen to amount to an agenda to deprive the father of the research evidence about the birth experience. In a later chapter, this selective truth-telling is referred to as a 'Conspiracy of silence' (See Chapter 8), much to the chagrin of the men on the receiving end who are prepared to articulate it. The role of the print media as well as the electronic media should not be underestimated here. It may be that the efforts of the press, combined with those of 'new fathers' such as David Beckham and the Prince of Wales, have not served to benefit the more standard form of father.

Another example of the electronic media role in the creation of the 'new father' is found in the website of Fathers Direct (2002). This ambiguously named organisation claims in its website that its mission :'exists to promote close and positive relationships between men and their children.' There are frequent mentions by Fathers Direct of the father's responsibility. There is, however, no indication of whether anybody, other than the father, is likely to benefit from the existence of this organisation. It may be surprising to some of us to find that the children of the fathers are not actually mentioned and that the mother is only mentioned in a disparaging way. Yet again, it would appear that the media are providing a less than completely balanced picture of parenthood.

The argument

The topic of this book has engendered considerable hilarity in some of the men with whom I have been able to discuss it. Their mirth arises from their need to emphasise the man's crucial contribution at the time of the conception. One example came to me in the form of a personal anecdote:

MIDWIFE: Would you like to be with your wife at the birth, Mr Jones?
MR JONES: Why would I want to do that? As long as I was there at the conception I'm happy.

By way of an introduction to the argument, I would like to contemplate briefly the reasons underpinning this humorous ribaldry. I consider here whether, as is so often the case, such humour has a more serious side. It is necessary to contemplate whether such amusement represents a coping mechanism and, if so, why it is necessary.

Genealogy

In some ways the recognition of the physical fact of motherhood is easy. You might even say that it is obvious. Almost invariably the woman shows abdominal enlargement and ultimately she gives birth to a baby. What is usually patently obvious to any observer is that the woman is pregnant, that she experiences labour and that the baby emerges from her body during the process of the birth.

Fatherhood is not at all like that. The changes that the father experiences are not visible. In most societies there is only one stage in the childbearing process in which the father is actively and crucially involved. That stage is the conception and it is ordinarily a quite private matter.

The lack of visibility of fatherhood has given rise to concerns. In certain situations, especially historically among the nobility, 'precautions' have been taken around the time of the nuptials in order to ensure that the father is actually the father (Harris, 1984). The need for these 'precautions', however, does not feature among lesser mortals. The need for such 'precautions' among nobility relates to the prestigious inheritance which is likely to be involved, but their existence reflects a range of doubts and anxieties which are not unique to the upper echelons of society. Some of these doubts and anxieties relate to the child's paternity. Because the man is not always expected to be monogamous, he may fear that his partner may be similarly unfaithful. Thus a man is likely to become anxious that his partners' children may not necessarily be his. These traditional uncertainties of fatherhood are reflected in the old adage that: It's a wise child that knows its own father.

Such uncertainties have been exacerbated and developed into modern concerns by the recent advances in assisted reproductive technology. Through these techniques the role of the father may have been further reduced to that of little more than a 'stallion' (Stanway, 1984). In addition, the interventions involved in such technology are undertaken, not by a female partner who might ordinarily be accused of adultery, but by a member of a male-dominated profession. Thus the insult to the paternal self-esteem is likely to be compounded further.

History

The man's assumption of a dominant role in the physiological process of reproduction emerges in an old analogy. It may still be evident in some cultures which have recognised the link between sexual intercourse and the conception (Douglas, 1966: 191). The fact that in other cultures this analogy has been overtaken by scientific knowledge may be perceived as yet another blow to the man's self-esteem. The analogy is the perception that it is the male's 'seed' which is the uniquely active agent in the development of the human fetus and the baby (Ahern, 1978: 272; Jeffery and Jeffery, 1996: 19; Vincent-Priya, 1992). Through this logic the offspring is directly related only to the father, carrying only his characteristics through his genetic material. The woman in this scenario serves merely as the 'soil' into which the man's seed is deposited and which serves only to nourish that seed. The function of her body is just to facilitate the development of the seed to its full potential, but she does not contribute any active components. This perception may not be unrelated to the patriarchal views of paternity which I have mentioned already. The invention of the microscope and the resulting increase in knowledge of the process of fertilisation clearly dealt a serious blow to such ideas of male supremacy.

As well as these long-standing views of the singular role of the man in reproduction and the more recent threats to this role, there is a further under-lying and immutable factor. This is the unique ability of the woman to bear children. This fact, which may appear too obvious to even mention, carries with it the inevitable consequence that the man is required to be totally dependent on a woman or women to achieve procreation and, thus, his stake in eternity. It may be interesting to contemplate whether this dependence, or even impotence, has had any effects on the man's wish for involvement in the processes of childbearing.

Exclusion

The involvement of the man in childbirth has long and extensively been taboo. The rationale for this prohibition is not entirely certain. A number of factors may have been involved, the most obvious being the knowledge base. As long as care during labour was determined solely by the attendant's personal experience of childbearing, it was inevitable that only women would be in a position to provide such care (Tew, 1995: 41).

Second, the concept of adultery, which has been mentioned already, may be related to the woman being regarded as her husband's property. This applied particularly to her reproductive functions as represented by her reproductive organs (Towler and Bramall, 1986: 29). Thus, it would be logical for a husband to place a veto on a man's attendance at the birth.

The third factor is one that continues to exist in many cultures, but which may be difficult for a woman and for a midwife to comprehend. This is the concept of 'pollution' which has resulted in childbirth becoming 'an unclean subject, fit only for midwives and sow gelders' (Graham, 1969). This concept is not easy to understand in a supposedly sophisticated society, since it features certain quite distinct component parts. As the word 'pollution' and the quote (above) indicate, there is an element of uncleanness. This is prob-ably comparable with current media-hyped anxieties about blood-borne infectious diseases. It resulted in the low status of the midwife indicated in the quotation and also her continuing low status in certain modern cultures (Jeffery and Jeffery, 1996).

The other element of pollution is even more challenging, because it features supernatural phenomena. These phenomena may be deemed to be super-natural because the birth of a child almost inevitably involves bleeding. Unlike the bleeding caused by a traumatic wound, however, the bleeding of healthy childbirth is controlled physiologically and ceases spontaneously. The result is that, contrary to what happens to men and in nature, the woman does not die. Such bleeding has long been incomprehensible to men, who tend to assume that death inevitably follows the loss of blood.

The only possible explanation was that some form of mystical agency was involved in the birth. This agency could constitute a danger to men as much as a benefit. For these reasons the birthing woman (like her menstruating sister) was and may still be secluded and prohibited from a wide range of activities for fear of the dire consequences to the direct and indirect contacts (Frazer, 1922; Shorter, 1983). This line of thought has not only personal, but also policy implications. This was apparent in the essentially pronatalist authorities in many European countries, who were hampered in their efforts to boost the birth rate prior to 1900 by 'profound suspiciousness about the pregnant woman's power to contaminate the world about her' (Shorter, 1983: 288).

As Martin (1987: 97) discusses, however, such masculine 'suspiciousness' and the resulting vetoes were not without benefit to the childbearing or menstruating woman. The vetoes usually involved prohibition from performing some tediously menial form of food preparation and 'could very easily be perceived as providing a woman with a welcome vacation' (1987: 98).

Thus superstitious fear and lack of relevant knowledge were initially responsible for the man not being permitted to be present at or involved in the birth. These factors were reinforced by, first, the low status of midwives and, second, potentially hostile patriarchal power which for centuries deterred the man from seeking to provide care routinely (Carter and Duriez, 1986: 60). Two factors ultimately needed to converge to change this situation. It was necessary for the development of fashion to combine with the advent of medical learning to overcome the long-standing and profound resistance to the man's involvement in childbirth (Loudon, 1992: 167).

Recent history

Against this historical backdrop the man-midwife first began to be involved in healthy childbearing (see Chapter 1). He was soon followed by the obstetrician in the mid-nineteenth century (Carter and Duriez, 1986: 77). By the latter part of the twentieth century the man who was the father was successful in pursuing his medical brothers into the birthing room. Although the ingress of each of these men was hotly debated at the time, these changes have not been subjected to considered and objective reflection. Thus this book aims to focus on the research evidence and other literature in order to document the changes associated with the man's increasing involvement in childbearing. The focus will reflect the many widely accepted benefits of the man's involvement in childbirth and will attempt to both frame and answer the question of whether there may also be disadvantages.

As well as the genealogical, historical and supposedly unclean aspects of birth, there exists another aspect which may not be unrelated to those already mentioned. This is men's underlying fear that, at the birth, women are doing something that men are unable to do and from which they have traditionally been excluded. Perhaps the man does not really seek involvement, but neither does he wish to be excluded on terms that are not of his own making.

Chapter 1

Cultures and times

Introduction

In order to be able to describe the role of the man in childbirth it may be helpful to go back to our roots. This resonates with the old adage 'If you want to know the way forward, you must know where you've come from'. In this chapter the aim is to examine where the society of which we are members has come from in this respect. Thus this chapter comprises, first, an analysis of relevant cross-cultural issues. These issues will lead into an assessment of the literature on the history of the man in childbearing. By using these complementary approaches it will be possible to show why the man has traditionally been, and in many societies still is, excluded from childbearing related matters. This material will guide us to consider the series of events which, in modern Western society, have permitted this exclusion to be, not merely abandoned, but to actually be reversed.

Other societies

A cross-cultural approach will provide a pathway to facilitate understanding of the processes which influence attitudes to the role of the man in childbirth. Such an approach has been described by Laderman as 'invaluable in assessing questions of universality and validity of current Western concepts and practices' (1988: 86). She goes on to emphasise the way in which people have a tendency to take for granted the practices that are current in their locality. Such complacency is compounded by assumptions that local practices are standard, innate and sensible to the point of being inevitable. Thus, in this section, the intention is not merely to show the wide range of differing practices which pertain, but to use this material to shed light on the attitudes and behaviours that are so commonplace that they are likely to pass unnoticed. This section draws largely on anthropological material. The convention in that science, however, of focusing on individual ethnic groups is constrained here by the need for brevity. Thus, certain generalisations may be necessary. Further, in considering the attitudes prevalent in different societies, it is crucial to bear in mind the dynamic nature of those societies. Inevitably any society features ongoing change and development. This means that different individuals in that society are likely to occupy different points on the continuum of change (Woollett and Dosanjh-Matwala, 1990). Again, generalisations may appear which may not be accurate.

Presenting symptoms

As has been mentioned already (see above, Introduction), unlike his woman partner, the man shows no visible sign that he is going through the process of becoming a father. In Western society a woman's pregnancy is likely to carry with it certain privileges, such as the woman being excused from some social obligations. For example, at a celebration or office function a woman who is obviously pregnant would be unlikely to be questioned about why she refuses to drink alcohol. Any change in her male partner's behaviour, however, is likely to be noted with interest, concern or even disdain.

In other societies pregnancy may be viewed differently, but in the West pregnancy is likely to engender friendly curiosity. This interest may be found to be supportive by the pregnant woman. Such support would not be available to any male partner, simply by virtue of the fact that his impending fatherhood is not visible to the naked eye. Thus a potential source of helpful support is denied to him.

Against this background of the invisibility of forthcoming fatherhood, the man has been found to manifest a range of symptoms and behaviours. Thus, the man 'presents' his changing state in ways which, either spontaneously or through custom and practice, are considered to be culturally appropriate. This presentation, which has attracted considerable research and other attention, has become widely known as 'couvade'. This term is derived from the Old French verb 'couver', meaning to cover a nest of eggs in order to help them to hatch into chicks. The term was first applied to the human male by Tylor, an anthropologist, in 1865 when the new science of anthropology was just beginning to develop. Couvade is sometimes interpreted as meaning a 'sympathetic pregnancy' (About, 2002). In its relatively short history, the term 'couvade' has assumed or has been assigned a number of meanings, which may reflect the increasing interest in the man's participation in childbearing.

When it was first introduced, the term 'couvade' was used to refer to the ritual behaviours of the man around the time of the birth and shortly afterwards. An example of this meaning is found in the work of Mead and Newton (1967: 190) who describe the restriction of activities and 'regulation' of behaviours that are found in a wide range of 'primitive' peoples shortly after the birth. These behaviours were observed in peoples with beliefs in the power of magic or those who had only recently moved from a matrilineal society to one that was patrilineal (Dixon, 2000).

Subsequently, the terminology was appropriated by psychiatrists who sought to explain the male partner's symptoms which were interpreted as mimicking the pregnant woman's 'minor disorders of pregnancy'. The psychiatrists recategorised the concept of couvade by subdividing it. They renamed the original form '*ritual* couvade', and the newly described condition 'couvade *syndrome*' (Trethowan and Conlon, 1965).

Another reinvention of couvade syndrome was by a group of psychoanalysts; in this context it was used as evidence of male parturition envy (Bettelheim, 1954). The example which they use is the one that features in the fairy-story of 'Little Red Riding Hood'. Even more recently, a sociological explanation of couvade syndrome has been advanced. The argument in this discipline is that couvade is used to seek to address the perceived marginalisation of the father in childbearing (Summersgill, 1993).

While, for obvious reasons, couvade is generally viewed from a masculine viewpoint, Jacqueline Vincent-Priya (1992) provides a woman's eye-view. In her anthropological whistle-stop tour she describes the benefits of couvade to the pregnant woman. These advantages relate to the couvading man providing the pregnant woman with better support. Additionally, there may be a perception in the woman that the severity of his symptoms are a reflection of the depth of his affection for her. This perception is apparent in one Azark woman's proud boast: 'My man allus does my pukin' for me' (Vincent-Priya, 1992: 47).

Symptoms

As well as its varying interpretations, the manifestations of couvade syndrome have been described in a variety of different terms. It would appear that the one common factor in all of the descriptions of couvade syndrome is that, as Summersgill observes, the woman is invariably excluded (1993: 92). Originally ritual couvade, as it has become known, was described in terms of the man's behaviour at the time of and after the birth being comparable with the woman's. The man's preparations comprised, first and foremost, preparing for himself a suitably secluded environment. In addition, he abstained from sexual activity, he avoided potentially harmful or stimulating food and drink, and he ensured he took adequate rest. After the birth he would be cared for and would put the baby to his breast (Dixon, 2000). The care provided for the father could be by the new mother and he might even assume her place to the extent of wearing her clothes (Mason and Elwood, 1995). Thus, in these practices the basis becomes clear for McClain's (1982) suggestion that couvade may constitute a culturally approved method for resolving conflicts in the man's sexual identity.

A more recent study has demonstrated a more culturally relevant insight into couvade syndrome. Researchers in Wales have described couvade syndrome in terms of alterations in the man's health status (Thomas and

Upton, 2000). These researchers undertook a quantitative study using a structured questionnaire to examine the male partner's experiences and his responses and attitudes to impending fatherhood. Questionnaires were posted to 'all partners of women who were pregnant and attending a hospital antenatal clinic for the first time during a two month period' (Thomas and Upton, 2000: 218). As well as an attitude scale the questionnaire included a checklist of somatic or bodily symptoms, on which each of the men was asked to indicate which problems he had experienced since the onset of his partner's pregnancy.

Of the 52 per cent (n = 141) of the population who responded to the questionnaire, only 63 (44.7 per cent) men reported experiencing no symptoms of couvade syndrome. Among the remaining 78 men the number of symptoms experienced varied between one (in 20 men = 14.2 per cent) and six (in 6 men = 4.5 per cent). These researchers chose to define couvade syndrome as the presence of two or more relevant symptoms. By using this definition, 49 of the respondents (34.8 per cent) experienced couvade syndrome. The symptoms which were included in these researchers' checklist were (in descending order of frequency of reporting):

- Increased tiredness
- Increased stress
- Anxiety
- Inability to sleep
- Headaches
- Loss of appetite
- Weight gain
- Nausea/vomiting

(Thomas and Upton, 2000: 219)

These researchers identified a negative correlation between socio-economic class and the incidence of couvade syndrome, although the correlation was not strong enough to reach the level of significance. Thomas and Upton conclude that the incidence of couvade syndrome together with their anxiety, though not high, indicate that the psychosocial needs of the father are not being met. They go on to suggest that couvade syndrome should be renamed 'antenatal stress syndrome', in order to attract more appropriate attention for the father from health care personnel and other sources of support.

Unfortunately, the definition of couvade syndrome offered by Thomas and Upton (2000) is rather imprecise and it corresponds with the general preparations of the birthing environment included by Summersgill and contributing to his definition: 'Couvade . . . all behaviour associated with childbirth that involves the father giving up his normal routine activities and following new ritualised behaviour' (1993: 92).

Although Thomas and Upton supposedly focused on the more somatic forms of symptoms, their checklist features a large component of stress-related conditions. It would be invidious to suggest that the psychological symptoms reported by these researchers' respondents constitute 'ritualised behaviour'. This study may be further criticised on the grounds that there is no indication of the chronology of the appearance of symptoms. For this reason it is necessary to rely on the older work of Klein (1991) to identify the timing of the occurrence of couvade. This researcher identified a biphasic incidence. His study identified an onset of symptoms during the third month of pregnancy, followed by their disappearance and reappearance again shortly before term.

The significance of couvade

In the same way as the interpretation of the presentation of couvade has undergone a number of reincarnations (see pp. 11–12 above), so too has its significance changed over time. In their analysis of ritual couvade in 'primitive' peoples, Mead and Newton (1967) show how these behaviours create a role for the man in childbearing. These authors argue that fatherhood is a concept which does not occur naturally. They suggest that it is an artefact or a 'fundamental social invention' (1967: 189). To support their argument that ritual couvade assists the perpetuation of this artefact, they draw on evidence from anthropology and the culture of the twentieth-century American middle class.

The usual pattern of human parenting, according to Mead and Newton, is that the man makes provision for the children of whoever is his sexual partner at the time. This provision is made regardless of the children's biological origins. This providing role may be assumed by the state in highly organised societies, when a surrogacy arrangement pertains, through taxing the man in order to pay financial allowances to the mother.

In more 'primitive cultures', though, beliefs are widespread that the father's behaviour will affect the development of the fetus and child as much as anything which the mother does. Partly because of his potential to influence the child's health and partly because of his very variable exclusion or involvement in the birth process, couvade rituals have evolved to demonstrate his importance (Mead and Newton, 1967: 190). These authors go on to draw comparisons with American middle-class culture, where there is an emphasis, not on fatherhood, but on the wedding. This emphasis is associated, first, with the financial support of the family. The second reason is that, when these authors were writing, the American man was not involved with the birth; he was either totally excluded or had very restricted contact with the woman and child (Mead and Newton, 1967: 190). Thus, the couvade rituals were effectively brought forward in time to precede, hopefully, even the conception. Clearly the involvement of the man at the birth has moved on, but the rationale may still apply for the absence of ritual couvade around the time of the birth.

Issues

I have examined some aspects underpinning the phenomena which have, collectively, become known as couvade syndrome. I now attempt to identify the currently important issues. These issues serve to indicate some of the reasons why couvade is still significant in an industrialised society at the beginning of the twenty-first century.

The research interest aroused by couvade includes a large qualitative study by Dixon (2000). His study used oral history research methods. His data collection involved undertaking discursive interviews with 26 midwives and 25 fathers. In both groups he found that there was a wide age distribution and a wide range of backgrounds and experience. The main focus of Dixon's research was on the father's need to relate to the newborn infant.

Dixon's main finding was the paradoxical views of the two groups. These views contrasted markedly. This contrast manifested itself in the fathers being mainly concerned with their relationship with the newborn child, whereas the midwives perceived that the father was there to provide helpful support for his partner. Inadvertently, in spite of this, the midwives were found to be very adequately 'ministering' to the emotional needs of the new father. In this way, Dixon concluded, the midwives were unknowingly encouraging 'couvading' behaviours in the father. The father was thus able to express his psychosocial needs, and also the midwife was able to help him to meet those needs. Examples of this form of couvade emerged in two ways. The first was the multiplicity of supposedly 'small' activities which the midwife would ask the father to undertake. These included asking him to hold the woman's hand, give her sips of water, or mop her brow and face. As Midwife U observed of the fathers: 'They've taken part of our role, which is good' (Dixon, 2000: 281).

The further example of a way in which couvade manifested itself was in a highly specific and more *ritual* ritual; that is, the cutting of the umbilical cord by the father. This is an intervention which Dixon's midwife informants were keen to give as an example of the father's extending role. Dixon relates it in terms of its symbolism to the action of the Siriono people of Eastern Bolivia, for whom the cutting of the cord is a way of claiming paternity. He contends that this action is becoming a 'nascent ritual of modern child-birth' (2000: 281). The midwife informants in Dixon's study were unable to explain the origins of this practice. This fact may mean that cutting the cord is a true ritual in that it is undertaken more for its symbolic meaning than for any functional reason. It is interesting to note, though, that this ritual developed at a time when anxieties about infections borne by body fluids, including their splashing, were becoming more prominent. Summersgill

(1993: 93), on the other hand, is more scathing about the development of this ritual. He uses it as an example of condescending attitudes among maternity personnel. He argues that staff have patronisingly invented such 'token' actions for the father because of their inability to take him seriously. In spite of this, Dixon's research findings present a much more positive impression of the staff's acceptance of and the father's satisfaction with the couvade available to him in maternity units. Thus he concludes that this form of couvade is seen by all involved as facilitating the relationship between the father and baby, rather than just helping the father to cope with a challenging situation.

The historical development of couvade syndrome (Mason and Elwood, 1995) shows that the evidence relating to couvade is invariably socio-anthropological rather than physiological. Such evidence relates to the incidence, risk factors and psychoanalytical explanations of the man's symptoms. The behavioural aspects of couvade syndrome are interpreted by these authors as appropriate preparation for the man's impending father-hood. The plea by Mason and Elwood for a more biologically oriented study of couvade is based on the incidence of infanticide among a range of lower mammals. These authors attempt to argue that couvade syndrome is a hormonally determined precursor to effective parenting behaviour. The final trigger to such behaviour is his physical proximity to the woman approaching term. On this basis, a health intervention to prevent sub-optimal parenting is proposed as the ultimate benefit, although the feasibility of introducing such an intervention is difficult to assess.

Mason and Elwood's argument of the absence of a biophysiological model for couvade is more persuasive than their ultimate recommendation. Although it may not be these authors' intention, their argument showing the uncertain basis of couvade syndrome and, hence, fatherhood serves to support the contention advanced by Mead and Newton (above) that fatherhood is no more than a 'fundamental social invention' (1967: 189).

In another opinion piece, Summersgill (1993) also focuses on the local current place of couvade syndrome. He first regrets the limited attention paid to fatherhood and compares this unfavourably with the abundant attention which motherhood receives. This neglect is regarded as a form of marginal-isation of both the father and fatherhood. Summersgill develops his argument to suggest that the lack of interest in the father leads him, in turn, to feel that he should lack interest in parenting. In this way, a self-fulfilling prophecy will have been created. This is supported by the widespread view that the father has no real role between the conception and the baby being brought home. Against this rather bleak background, Summersgill suggests that the father becomes acutely aware of the pregnancy-related changes in his partner. In response, he 'adopts' (1993: 95) the symptoms which he has observed in her, to help him to cope with both his transition to fatherhood and her transition to motherhood.

The argument emerges that the underlying problem of new fatherhood is the lack of any formalised ritual couvade. Summersgill proposes that new forms of couvade may have been introduced, such as home improvement or 'DIY', or surfing the net for relevant research evidence or 'technology watching'. These new rituals, however, have not supplanted the more long-standing and meaningful couvade rituals. Thus the father is destined to remain in this marginalised limbo. Such a dismal scenario does not appear to be amenable to easy solutions. Perhaps inadvertently, though, Summersgill raises the question of why the father, in spite of his marginalisation, should choose to accompany the woman during childbirth. I would venture to argue that this question needs to be extended to include some consideration of who it is who is intended to benefit from his presence.

An answer to the latter question may be found in an anthropological study of the men of Karembola in southern Madagascar (Middleton, 2000). This researcher describes a Karembola man who is practising couvade by gathering herbs, preparing his wife's food and making himself unattractive to other women to avoid sex. His intention is to assert his involvement with the recent birth of his daughter. Middleton maintains that this man's behaviour is a demonstration of his paternity, which is intended to contrast with the claims of the 'ownership' of childbearing by women. In this way couvade may be seen to involve daily routines which have been subjected to gender reversal. The Karembola man could accurately be described as 'mothering the mother and baby in his house' (2000: 118) with the intention of proving that women do not have the monopoly on birth. This man is therefore seeking to assert his authority or control over a situation, new fatherhood, which otherwise verges on the uncontrollable.

This examination of the issues relating to ritual couvade and couvade syndrome shows that couvade is indubitably about the balance of power in childbearing. In the next section the importance of power relations surfaces again in a cross-cultural setting through an examination of the concept of pollution.

Pollution

I have suggested that couvade practices may be the man's method of assuming some control over his partner's childbearing experience. Similarly, the concept of pollution may reflect a society's control or power over some of its members. This concept is of additional significance in relation to men and childbearing because pollution is likely to be one of the reasons why, in many traditional societies, men have avoided becoming involved with childbearing. In considering pollution, what emerges as crucial is the relationship between the society in its broadest terms and the individuals who make up that society. In the manifestations and control of pollution the actions and behaviours of the society and its members have powerful implications for each other.

The concept of pollution has been shown to exist more or less explicitly in many former and current cultures. Because of the differing contexts, although it has invariably featured certain specific characteristics, pollution may be known by a number of alternative names. It was the term 'pollution' which featured in the title of the influential book by Douglas (1966). 'Impurity' was the word used by Rozario (1992), since her focus was more on the society as opposed to the individuals who were its members. Mead and Newton (1967), who concentrated on the pathologically negative aspects of this concept, chose to refer to its 'defiling' nature. The full implications of this concept were brought home to me when working with a highly articulate and devout woman who was a member of the South Asian community in Scotland. She was grieving the death of her newborn daughter who had had serious cardiac problems. During our conversation she mentioned that her grief was not helped by her inability to find comfort in her Koran or to attend her baby's funeral; both were forbidden her due to her 'unclean' state. Like me, my midwife colleagues also found some difficulty understanding this grieving mother's sad predicament.

Rationale

The assumptions underlying the concept of pollution are spelt out by Ahern who writes about the experience of Chinese women (1978: 271). She observes that any fluid or other substance which escapes from the body is automatically assumed to be unclean. This observation applies to material which escapes from any of the orifices, regardless of the state of the person's health. Particularly polluting, according to Rozario writing in the context of southern Asia (1992: 99), are the fluids associated with four bodily processes: sexual intercourse, menstruation, childbirth and breast-feeding.

The differential production of these four fluids is regarded as the crucial difference in the relative purity of the woman and the man. The man is perceived as being relatively pure because male pollution is controllable, on account of the production of male sexual fluids being controllable by celibacy. Further, Douglas (1966: 3) emphasises how each sex's reproductive and sexual fluids are perceived as being especially dangerous to the other sex. In spite of this, the man's vulnerability to the woman's sexual fluids is regarded as a more serious problem. So, although there may appear to be a balance or symmetry between the sexes, this is not actually the case. The situation is that a hierarchy exists in terms of the man's greater vulnerability and the woman being more dangerous. As well as the fluids representing different levels of impurity, the production of the fluids also renders the woman more dangerous. This is partly because, unlike the man, female pollution is not controllable by celibacy, as the woman sheds blood vaginally during menstruation unless she is pregnant. In addition, the fact that the woman produces fluids associated with all four of the bodily processes, rather than only one like the man, aggravates her impure state (Rozario, 1992: 99).

Further, the woman is considered to be uniquely polluting because of the blood which she loses during menstruation and childbirth. Blood carries a multiplicity of levels of significance in relation to pollution. Essentially blood is indubitably good and beneficent while circulating through the blood-vessels. When it is lost vaginally, however, it becomes absolutely evil and dirty (Ahern, 1978: 271). The harmful properties of menstrual blood feature prominently in 'virtually every society on record'. The dangerousness of blood tends to prevent the woman from doing her work due to detrimental effects on, for example, wine, meat, bread, preserves and infants (Shorter, 1983: 287).

Menstrual blood is held to be destructive because, originating supposedly as part of the embryo, its shedding may be construed as murder of the embryo (Rozario, 1992: 98). This South Asian view is endorsed among Chinese communities, who ascribe menstrual blood's dangerous properties to it being made up of a part of the child's 'soul' (Ahern, 1978: 272). Menstrual blood may even be given the status of a dead person, on the grounds that it had the potential to become a human being. If the blood had not flowed, the argument goes, a child would have been born (Douglas, 1966: 96).

Thus, during menstruation and childbirth, the woman's polluting nature reduces her status to being at the lowest level of society – that of the 'untouchables'. Menstrual blood and lochia (the blood which is shed vaginally after the birth) may be thought to be the same fluid, as menstrual fluids are said to collect in the womb during pregnancy. Birth fluids are considered dirtiest of all the bodily fluids, due to their nature, quantity and the duration of their production. The polluting nature of these fluids is considered to be comparable with the fluids of the dead body in terms of the danger which they have the propensity to exert (Douglas, 1966: 34).

The collection of menstrual fluid in the womb during pregnancy may be thought to represent a considerable danger to those nearby. For this reason, Shorter reports, pregnant women have been excluded from religious and other celebrations, especially those involving children and young people (1983: 288). The dirty or defiling condition associated with the birth begins as soon as the labour starts (Mead and Newton, 1967: 174). The impurity is sufficiently dangerous for the Arapesh woman to have to give birth on the edge of the village in the 'bad place' which is kept for excretion, menstrual huts and pigs. The birth fluids are similar in their dangerousness to menstrual fluids, but with the added property of (if damaged) being able to harm the newborn (Ahern, 1978: 272). All of the negative properties of menstrual fluid are also inherent in the lochia.

The pollution associated with childbirth is sufficiently serious for it to be comparable with the pollution of death. This comparison may be quite apposite in view of the risk of mortality which childbirth may carry (King, 1983: 121). Douglas argues, however, that although both are seriously polluting: 'Pollution resulting from childbirth is milder than the pollution consequent on death' (1966: 66). As well as the risk of contagion and contamination carried by the birth fluids, the woman and any birth companions are subject to supernatural influences. This is because birth is regarded as a time when the woman and the baby are vulnerable to death. Thus the risk of supernatural or demoniacal forces applies both during as well as after the birth. For this reason, a 'lying in' period may be recommended to resist these evil influences (Mead and Newton, 1967: 175).

Pollution is not necessarily an absolute, in that different levels of seriousness of pollution may be identified. An example of this debate has been mentioned already, relating to whether childbirth or death is the more polluting.

Significance of pollution

The significance of pollution, as has been indicated above, varies between different ethnic groups. Rozario compares the different interpretations between Hindu and Islamic peoples (1992: 98). She concludes that Islamic beliefs are less extreme than those of Hindus. She observes further that, in Islam, women are not the only stigmatised group but that prohibitions may apply equally to prohibited and polluted males. The effect of pollution in 'primitive' religions is examined by Douglas (1966: 1), who finds that impurity, defilement and poor hygiene raise fear and dread among devotees. She goes on to emphasise, though, that such beliefs are not unique to 'primitives'. Early Christians objected strongly to pollution by blood as well as to conditions such as leprosy. Douglas quotes Archbishop Theodore of Canterbury (668–90), who required women to undergo 40 days of purgation after childbirth. Further he exacted a penance of three weeks' fasting for a woman (lay or religious) who entered the church or took communion while menstruating (1966: 60); the infamous practice of some Christian sects of 'churching of women' after childbirth is clearly not unrelated. Although this ceremony is said to be interpreted only as a form of thanksgiving, a woman in a recent research project found it to be necessary for her after giving birth (Mander, 1995). Rozario builds on this Christian interpretation of the significance of pollution by showing how closely it corresponds with that religion's concept of sin (1992: 98). She develops this argument by suggesting that all societies incorporate social hierarchies which parallel the dogma of purity/impurity; further, social distancing may be created on even flimsier bases, such as by the strictures of dress, manners or etiquette.

A significant issue which this examination of pollution brings to our attention is the problem of the marginal states. This marginality applies to people who are not included in the patterning of society and who are considered, for this reason, to be 'placeless' (Douglas, 1966: 95). Marginality is most readily apparent in the unborn child who is thus regarded as being both vulnerable and dangerous. Because the fetus is so demanding of available resources to ensure its growth and survival, the pregnant woman, to satisfy those demands, also becomes dangerous. A range of susceptible people, such as those who are unwell or undergoing some life transition, are also vulnerable to and capable of exerting this form of danger.

Although writing about their work in South Asia, Jeffery and her colleagues emphasise the universality of the concept of childbirth pollution (1989: 124). These researchers liken pollution to power, in that unless power is used properly or is controlled it has the potential to become evil. In the same way the woman and her baby are capable of harming or defiling other people but they are simultaneously vulnerable. Thus in order to protect both the mother and baby dyad and those who are nearby, isolation and purification rituals are necessary. Jeffery and colleagues quote five weeks as the maximum period of seclusion, which equates with 1.25 months or 40 days. The period of isolation is intended to continue for as long as the woman's impurity or lochial discharge. In spite of this dogma, in practice there is a gradual resumption of the woman's usual activities.

The group among whom pollution achieves its major significance is within the family or the extended family – the caste. Rozario maintains that the purity or impurity of the women in the group determines the honour and status of the men and, hence, of the family or caste (1992: 98). She goes on to show how anxiety about the women's pollution or purity results in the men's preoccupation with control over women. This preoccupation results in child marriage and widow burning (*sati*), as the purity of a woman can be maintained or ensured only by her being overseen by a husband. In this way direct connections become apparent between sexuality, pollution, purity of the caste (as represented by the bloodline) and masculine control over women. Rozario continues by showing how, if impure, the woman is regarded as powerful, whereas purity is associated with an absence of power and the need for protection. Thus, the power of the masculine role is further enhanced.

Symbolism

As well as its practical importance, pollution is also significant because of its multiplicity of symbolic meanings. The primary symbolism of pollution relates to the crucial transitions in the life cycle with which it is associated. The transitions which happen throughout life represent threats to the composure and, perhaps, the integrity of the individual. These threats manifest themselves most obviously during adolescence, following a bereavement and around the time of the birth. Such transitions may be viewed as margins or as thresholds to a new lifestyle and, as such, they may be perceived as dangerous. It may be helpful to think of the healthy body symbolically as representing an orderly society. Even in health the margins of the body are where the uncertainties and threats to that order lurk. To continue the analogy with the body, the margins are represented by the orifices. It is from these openings that substances which are deemed to be dangerous may emanate and, reciprocally, other agents which are dangerous to the body may gain entry. Thus, symbolically, the orifices are perceived as the vulnerable and dangerous points both in the body and in the society (Douglas, 1996: 114). On this basis, it is logical that the vaginal bleeding following the birth of a child, with exposure to the associated risk of death at the time of the transition to motherhood, should be regarded as supremely dangerous (King, 1983: 121).

The symbolic role of the woman is regarded as being to act as the keeper of the gate by which entry is gained into the family or caste. This is an immense responsibility, since the effectiveness of this role determines the continuing purity or otherwise of the patrilineal family line. Laxity in the woman's sexual behaviour or in her observance of ritual may be perceived as a threat to far more than those who are in direct contact with her. These are threats because the orderliness of the society may be at stake through the agency of the woman and the fluids which escape from her body during and following the birth.

Writing in the context of the traditional Chinese family, Ahern (1978: 275) considers the power and the danger in the woman's social and reproductive roles. The role of the married woman is perceived by her husband's family as being to produce sons who will make offerings to the gods when the husband's parents die. This woman, though, is regarded as a very mixed blessing. There may be suspicions that she will form affectionate bonds with her children in order to secure some advantage in her own old age. In this way the wife may be seen as an intruder into her husband's family. Her self-seeking activities may undermine her husband's authority in her attempts to make her own way. Chinese men think along these lines, leading to suspicion that the young woman may subvert and, hence, disrupt the cohesiveness of the family. Such disruption is dangerous, as the stability and continuation of the family line are of prime importance. It is not difficult to envisage that these perceptions and activities are likely to engender disharmony due to the underlying mistrust of the young wife's ambiguously powerful position in the family.

Again it emerges, through its symbolism, that the relative balance of power between the man and the woman in the more or less extended family is fundamental to the concept of pollution.

Manifestations

Passing reference has been made to some of the ways in which the existence of pollution may manifest itself. The taboos which are commonly applied during periods of pollution are well known. In the UK it is not so long since a mother would forbid her young daughter to wash her hair during her menstrual period. Similarly, the taboo on sexual intercourse during the puerperium may still exist (Hawkins and Higgins, 1981: 393). Shorter (1983: 288) outlines some of the fearful consequences which may befall the new mother in some European countries should she ignore and break the taboos on her activities.

The new mother may be secluded or undergo a period of isolation in order to reduce the risk of her contaminating others who may be vulnerable (Vincent-Priya, 1992: 113). Such prohibition is likely to apply to the woman's husband as much as to any other man and certainly to any form of sexual contact (Mead and Newton, 1967: 173). The period of the new mother's seclusion is prescribed and ends with a purification ritual, such as a special bath (Jeffery *et al.*, 1989: 124). These rituals are likely to involve people other than just the woman. Shorter emphasises that the public nature of these ceremonies serves to impress on the other members of the society the risks which may accrue to them if such observances are not followed (1983: 289).

Implications

The ritual aspects of pollution illustrate to others, who are not directly involved, the significance of the change in the person's status. As well as driving home the message of the risk of contamination, outsiders are made to realise that the polluted woman is or has been a danger as much to herself as to other people. Douglas cites the work of Van Gennep (1960) in which he explored the dangers inherent in these marginal states, and which may be compared with the betwixt and between nature of the corridors of a house. The change in the person's status may involve being a temporary outcast from the society. In the case of the new mother this is likely to take the form of social exclusion from the usual activities of the family group.

The social function of the concept of pollution emerges as being indubitably more significant than its health function. One of the ways in which this operates is through the ordering of the social group with well-defined structures. Crucial to the concept of pollution is 'dirt', which Douglas defines as simply being 'matter out of place' (1966: 35). She expands this definition to recount how dirt offends against the orderliness of the society. The efforts to remove or control dirt through pollution precautions constitute attempts to organise the social environment. Douglas indicates, however, that it is not only the reality of dirt which threatens the social order. It is also disobedience to the rules and rituals which control the perception of dirt and, thus, maintain a pure or unpolluted state. Ahern builds on Douglas' argument by emphasising that it is the *male* social order which is under threat (1978: 277). Disobedience to conventions may be in the form of deliberate misbehaviour or by inadvertently ignoring certain rituals, which may cause the development of impurity.

The orderliness of the status quo may be interpreted in two ways, which may be linked. The first, more obvious, aspect relates to the individuals' wealth. Rozario (1992) contends that purity is more easily achieved by the wealthy. This is presumably due to their vested interest in maintaining a stable, orderly society; any questioning of financial inequalities would inevitably carry risks of disorder.

This link between purity and higher social status leads into the second aspect, which is the different roles of women and men. In a society in which rulings are made by the eldest male in the family, a young woman is likely to be blamed for causing social disorder or 'disharmony' if and when she decides not to follow those rulings (Ahern, 1978: 276). In more general terms, assumptions may be made by a male-dominated society that the woman is impure and the man is pure (Rozario, 1992: 102). Although more explicit in some societies, female sexual purity is crucial to all of the major religions and, as has been argued above, the need for such purity may be traced back to the honour, status and reputation of a patrilineal elite. In this debate women are inevitably inferior and less powerful and are therefore the oppressed group. Thus, the concept of pollution is used to maintain the status quo by reinforcing existing social pressures.

In summary, the literature shows that the concept of pollution has been widely employed to maintain a balance of power between women and men, which indisputably advantages the latter. This concept is based on an assumption of the dangerously evil nature of women at certain well-defined times in their lives and, possibly, more generally. Having shown the low esteem in which the childbearing woman and her experience may be held, it is now appropriate to consider the role of the person who attends the woman in childbirth in cultures where the concept of pollution features prominently and explicitly.

The attendant at the birth

While the birth attendant may be regarded as occupying a marginal status even in sophisticated societies, her situation is even more uncertain where pollution features. If the concept of pollution predominates in a culture, the status of the person who attends the birth is likely to be beneath contempt. A well-researched example of this role is that of the *dai* in South Asia (Jeffery *et al.*, 1989). The woman who takes up this work is likely to do so for the lack of any other form of financial support. According to Jeffery and colleagues (1989: 68), the *dai* is usually an older woman who has been widowed, has no sons or who is unsupported for some other reason. Her lowly occupation effectively causes her to be totally ostracised from social contacts and even from her own family. The *dai* is despised, not only by the menfolk, but also by the childbearing women who call on her services to assist at the birth. The words of the *dai* imply that she may even despise herself:

> 'How can I think this work is good or bad since I do it out of necessity? I have to do it.'

'I work as a *dai* out of necessity. Would I do this work . . . if we owned land?'

(Jeffery et al., 1989: 65)

The birth attendant in history

This brief mention of the attitudes of non-Western societies to the processes around the time of the birth provides an indication of why certain groups have chosen not to be present at the birth of a baby. This examination leads logically to the low-status birth attendant who has been treated as a pariah, outcast or untouchable in her own community. Having considered the reasons for choosing not to be involved, it is now appropriate to examine who actually undertook this work. It is necessary to bear in mind that such work has long carried the potential to alienate the person from the other members of her (or possibly his) community.

The womenfolk

Since human beings began to congregate in communities, women have come together when a birth is imminent (Towler and Bramall, 1986: 3). This coming together still features in some non-Western communities, such as in Northern India, where Jeffery and colleagues observed: 'During labour, most women are with at least a couple of other women who stay throughout' (1989: 100).

This supportive arrangement has also been recorded in early Western societies. Kitzinger (1994) maintains that historically other women came to be with and to help a woman both during and after childbirth. These women were family, in-laws, neighbours and friends. They were known as the 'god-siblings', god-sibs or gossips, meaning the woman's sisters in God, due to their role at the child's baptism (Davis-Floyd and Sargent, 1997). Wilson details the processes involved in collecting the god-sibs together in seventeenth- and eighteenth-century East Anglia. He reports that virtually the only role for the father was 'nidgeting' (1995: 25), which meant that the father went to the relevant houses to indicate that labour had begun and that the woman's company was being sought. Thereafter the father had no part to play in the proceedings. The labour and lying-in were very much a social event involving only women, during which time the new mother was supported, nurtured and encouraged by other women who had survived the experience of giving birth. The inevitable hostility of the menfolk to this all-female celebration resulted in the eventual change of meaning of 'gossips' to its current derogatory use.

As well as the gossips, the midwife would stay with the woman for the duration of the labour and birth. Wilson provides a clear picture of the relatively high social status of the woman who served as midwife. Regardless of her age and her social origins, the title of 'midwife' placed this woman in a superior role around the time of the birth. In addition, unlike the gossips, who received only their food and drink, the midwife was paid in cash for her attendance at the birth.

The situation which Wilson recounts as happening in East Anglia was the invariable arrangement for healthy birth in the British Isles up until the late sixteenth century. Childbearing was very much women's business (Barclay *et al.*, 1989). Whether men were actually excluded by the womenfolk or whether they chose to exclude themselves in order to avoid pollution is not entirely clear. Their role was limited, though, to peripheral activities, such as the 'nidgeting' mentioned by Wilson (1995: 25). During the month or 'her month' when the woman was 'lying in', the husband would have to do her usual work in addition to his own, such as carrying sacks of meal. The woman would be literally confined to her lying-in room and the only permissible visitors would be women. Thus, men were generally kept away and the only males who were permitted to visit would be close relatives.

The midwife was quite well able to manage any of the common problems which may arise in childbearing. If, however, the woman's labour became seriously prolonged to the point of obstruction and the fetus died, a barber-surgeon would be called by the midwife to remove the fetus piecemeal. The barber-surgeons were almost invariably men. In such a dire situation they would resort to the use of instruments such as hooks, levers, crotchets, fillets and perforators. The use of these instruments was forbidden to the midwife. The hope was that their use would save the mother's life (Carter and Duriez, 1986: 36).

There were some midwives, however, whose practice went beyond the usual non-interventive orientation. A good example of such a midwife was Sarah Stone, who practised around Taunton, where there was no barber-surgeon to provide help in an emergency (Wilson, 1995: 58). Effectively Sarah Stone undertook many of the manipulations which would have been made by a barber-surgeon had one been available. These operations, however, were completed in a midwifery; that is, a social and domestic context. The crucial difference was that, rather than using instruments which were forbidden to her to achieve her outcomes, she used her hands. In this way she was able to assist the birth of a live baby to a healthy mother, even after the labour was thought to have become obstructed.

The existence of expert midwives such as Sarah Stone does not alter the clear division of labour which pertained until at least the late sixteenth and early seventeenth centuries. At that time a series of highly significant developments occurred in close succession.

The entrance of men into the birthing room

In England a number of male-oriented developments occurred around the early part of the seventeenth century. These events had momentous implications for both the midwife and the woman for whom she provided care. These developments featured the entry of men into the birthing arena or even the birthing room and serve as examples of subsequent phenomena. In association with these events the nature of childbearing was changed utterly. Whereas birth had been women's business which was undertaken in a social setting in a domestic context, the arrival of men into the birthing sphere converted it into a scientific, pseudo-medical phenomenon with unlimited scope for intervention.

The Chamberlen dynasty

As well as their single major innovation, the Chamberlens demonstrate certain characteristics which may have persisted. They were a French Huguenot family with a singular lack of imagination in choosing the names of their children. Four generations of this dynasty oversaw the initiation of crucial and fundamental changes in the practice of midwifery. Seven male family members practised midwifery and surgery; in so doing they conspired to develop and profit maximally from the development of the midwifery (later obstetric) forceps (Wilson, 1995: 53). This family's behaviour may appear quite unethical by current standards. Aveling, however, excuses their actions on the grounds that keeping trade secrets for profit was standard practice for surgeons and physicians in the seventeenth and eighteenth centuries (1882).

THE FAMILY

The dynasty began with William Chamberlen and his wife Genevieve who, as Protestants, avoided the St Bartholomew's Day massacre in 1569 in Paris by fleeing to Southampton. They brought with them their small family of Peter, Simon and Jane. Their other son Peter, known as the younger, seems to have been born into the family about three years later. Although it is not certain, Aveling suggests that William Chamberlen may have been a medical practitioner (1882: 4).

Peter Chamberlen the elder became a barber-surgeon with a considerable 'midwifery' practice. This Peter proved to have difficulty accepting the authority of the college which supervised the barber-surgeons. He was not the only member of his dynasty to encounter this difficulty. He practised repeatedly outwith the scope of his barber-surgeon licence, by administering medicines for internal consumption. This was a practice permitted only to physicians. He was imprisoned for what appears to have been a rather arrogant attitude to authority and was released only through the intervention of powerful family members. It seems rather strange that the birth of Peter the younger was not recorded at the time, so that it needed to be certified by a deposition in 1596. Like his elder brother, Peter the younger missed lectures and was fined for misdemeanours. He became a barber-surgeon in 1596 and was subsequently licensed by the Bishop of London to practise midwifery. As well as coming into conflict with physicians, this 'insolent' young man irritated the guild board by allying himself with traditional female midwives to achieve their incorporation.

A still more flamboyant character, Dr Peter Chamberlen was the eldest son of Peter the younger. Dr Peter had become a medical practitioner by the age of 18, having been educated at the universities of Cambridge, Heidleberg and Padua. He was also in dispute with the guild board over his 'frivolous' mode of dress (Aveling, 1882: 35) and interprofessional transgressions. Like his father, Dr Peter sought unsuccessfully to assist the regulation of midwives. With his advancing years Dr Peter became an increasingly eccentric polymath, with a religious fanaticism which verged on mania.

The eldest son of Dr Peter was named Hugh. Although there are no records of a medical degree and because his eldest son had the same first name, he is known as Hugh Chamberlen the elder. As well as attempting unsuccessfully to sell the family secret of the midwifery forceps to Mauriceau in France, Hugh Chamberlen the elder translated Mauriceau's textbook into English with certain important additions. Like other members of his family, he was imprisoned for professional misconduct. After some financial adventures Hugh Chamberlen the elder retired to Holland where, according to Aveling (1882: 154), he eventually managed to sell the family secret.

Paul Chamberlen was the second son of Hugh Chamberlen the elder, but his midwifery practice and financial deals were less remarkable than his relatives'. John Chamberlen was, like his father Paul, not very noteworthy. Hugh Chamberlen the younger, apart from some interprofessional indiscretions, followed a relatively blameless midwifery career.

THE ISSUES

Certain themes emerge from the saga of this extraordinary family. As well as their difficulties with senior members of their own occupational group, the Chamberlens appear to have thrived on generating interprofessional conflict. This began with Peter the elder's being imprisoned for practising medicine without a licence to Hugh the younger setting himself up in competition with apothecaries. Of particular interest in this context, though, is the recurring relationship with the traditional female midwives. Peter the younger, acting philanthropically, according to Aveling (1882: 5), sought to better the midwife's lot by improving education leading to greater security. Even Aveling, however, is unable to excuse the political manoeuvring of Dr Peter Chamberlen by which he sought, and was recognised by the college of barber-surgeons, to try to establish a monopoly midwifery practice. This was to be achieved by his agreeing only to provide emergency attention to women in the care of the midwives who had 'confirmed' themselves to him.

In the course of these attempts he was accused of being both 'insolent' and 'boastful' (Aveling, 1882: 15). Following the traditional traits of the old professions, he further attempted to control his market by using financial sanctions. Not only did Dr Peter attend only rich clients after he had made demands for 'great reward' (Aveling, 1882: 34), but he also declined to attend the poor. Such questionably ethical behaviour did nothing to endear Dr Peter to the midwives, who made a complaint to the guild.

The absence of crucial documentation is interesting in a family which appears to have relied heavily on authentic records. This omission applies first to the birth records of Peter the younger and later to the medical qualifications of Hugh the elder.

In spite of the apologist stance assumed by Aveling (1882), the ethics of keeping secret a device, the midwifery forceps, which was supposed to be able to save the lives of babies and mothers, needs to be questioned. The entrepreneurial orientation of this family is clearly apparent, both in this matter and in the business dealings which accompanied their practice. This does not excuse such secrecy however, as the invention might have remained hidden indefinitely, but for the curiosity of a much later inhabitant of the Chamberlens' house.

The way that the forceps were kept secret when in use also merits attention. Dunn (1999) recounts the lengths to which the Chamberlens went to disguise or hide the nature of their intervention. These strategies included transporting the instruments in an oversized chest which could only be carried by two people. All family and other attendants were sent from the birthing room and the woman herself was blindfolded. Loud noises were produced by other means to disguise any sound made by the metal forceps. This device was clearly a trade secret, but the treatment of a labouring woman and concerned family in such a way was truly cavalier.

Hugh the elder's translation of Mauriceau's midwifery book matters here for two reasons. The first relates to the material which was translated. The French man-midwife was also in the business of seeking to enhance his income and he was not concerned whether this threatened the livelihood of the midwife. Thus, his book recommended that physicians should be involved in more births, even those which showed no sign of becoming complicated. Perhaps in support of this recommendation, Hugh the elder published certain claims to indicate the benefits of the involvement of a man-midwife. In his translation Hugh the elder claimed to be able to deliver the baby alive from a living mother even when labour had become obstructed. Such an intervention, he indicated, removed the need for destructive operations using instruments such as hooks. This secret, according to Hugh the elder, was known only to members of his family, and would certainly be of no use to midwives.

Even Aveling, writing almost two centuries later, was still describing the forceps in terms of their ability to save lives. Unfortunately, there was a tendency to ignore the potential for damage to many more. Loudon reinforces this warning, stating that while forceps were advantageous in that they reduced the need for destructive instruments, their main strength was that until about 1860 physicians tended to be 'very – even excessively – conservative in their use' (1882: 19).

This brief examination of the role of the Chamberlen dynasty shows that their introduction of the midwifery forceps was, to be generous, questionably ethical. It would not be an understatement to suggest that these four generations of one family were largely responsible for the move of childbearing out of the domestic sphere where women were responsible for their own and each other's care into the hands of men.

William Harvey

The childbearing implications of William Harvey's work operate at a number of levels and at varying degrees of complexity. Harvey was born in Kent in 1578 and died in 1657, having travelled widely, but he completed his most influential work in London. Undoubtedly Harvey's major contribution to knowledge was the discovery of the role of the heart and the circulation of the blood. This discovery was based on his animal experiments, his human dissections and his understanding of the ancient scholars, particularly Aristotle (Cunningham, 2002).

As well as its general relevance, Harvey's work is significant here for his introduction of science to the study of anatomy. Previous knowledge and practice had been based on the work of Galen and Aristotle. The long-held belief was that there were two compartments of blood in the body, each having crucially different features and functions. Harvey's discovery contradicted traditional thought and called into question centuries of physicians' practice. Not surprisingly, his publication, *De motu cordis* (1628), engendered fierce opposition (Keele, 1965).

Jean Riolan the younger, an academic anatomist in Paris, was particularly vocal in opposing Harvey. As well as influential opponents, however, there were many enthusiasts for Harvey's ideas, particularly in Central Europe. A fellow countryman of Riolan, René Descartes (1596–1650), did not just accept the concept of the circulation of the blood; he modified it to build his own doctrine published as *Discourse on Method* in 1637. Descartes sought anatomical and physiological explanations of all the phenomena which are characteristic of the human body. Employing the newly developing scientific method to find them, he embraced Harvey's account of the circulation with enthusiasm. By the use of both dissection and introspection Descartes was coming to regard the human body no longer as the sacred temple of the soul, but as a mundane machine controlled by physical principles (Melzack, 1993). Harvey was dismayed to find that his ideas were being manipulated to support a theory of automatic, self-regulating systems. Cartesian ideas view the body as a machine, which needs only mechanical interventions by artisans to remedy problems. These ideas have continued to determine knowledge and therapy and may still persist. Cartesian duality, which separates the 'human spirit' from the physical body, may be associated with the well-known stereotypes of masculine objectivity.

The scientific ideas of Harvey and Descartes were applied to childbearing by a Scotsman, William Smellie (1697–1763). Following nineteen years of general practice in rural Lanarkshire, Smellie travelled to London in order to increase his knowledge and improve his practice (Willocks, 1986). Smellie's study of the processes of labour and childbirth produced two major outcomes. The first was the less than balanced, yet understandable, hostility of the midwife Mrs Elizabeth Nihell. Her vehement opposition to and ridicule of him and his instruments may have served to obscure the more insidious harm resulting from Smellie's other major achievement. This was his accurate and objective measurement of the woman's pelvis and his description of the way in which the fetus negotiates a way through it during labour and birth. While such measurements and descriptions are by definition value-free, the use to which they are put may be more disconcerting. In the same way as Descartes had effectively reduced the human body to a machine, Smellie reduced childbirth to a series of 'Powers, passages and passengers'. The human woman, with her emotions such as confidence and anxiety, was effectively being obliterated from childbirth. It may be that this obliteration was more insidiously damaging to women and their midwives than the invention and application of obstetric forceps by a man-midwife.

As well as Harvey's discovery having implications for the population as a whole, I have suggested that his 'scientific' approach was eventually associated with alterations in the care of the childbearing woman. These changes may have occurred in spite of Harvey's relatively cautious approach to childbirth expounded in his lesser known publication, *De Generatione*. This work focused mainly on the reproduction of lower animals, but recommendations were made for the care of the woman in labour. Although the work was completed at an earlier stage in Harvey's career, it was not published until 1651. Because of his advocacy of patience and watchfulness and his avoidance of the use of instruments, Harvey was named the 'Father of English Midwifery', although this was by the physician Percival Willoughby (Keele, 1965).

The modern male midwife

In historical terms, the emergence of the modern midwife who is a man is relatively recent. This person is very different from the man-midwife, such as William Smellie, mentioned above. The difference is that the man-midwife evolved from the barber-surgeon and eventually metamorphosed into the obstetrician. The male midwife, however, has a background, an education and occupational experience which is comparable with any midwife who is female.

One of the problems with which the male midwife must contend is his job title. In this context it is necessary to disregard those who are ignorant enough to think he should be styled 'mid-husband' (Dixon, 2000). It is argued quite appropriately that a person's gender should not determine his job title (Robotham, 1998: 63); this matters no more than his skin colour, age or religion. In spite of this statement of the obvious, the term 'male midwife' is widely used (Bahl, 1996; Catanzariti, 2001; O'Bryant, 2001; Robotham, 1998; Sanz, 2001; Speak and Aitken-Swan, 1982). Not least do these men themselves use the term. In his occasional publications on the topic, Lewis uses no other term (1989, 1991, 1998). Hence, mainly for the latter reason but also for its brevity, I use the term 'male midwife' here.

The phenomenon which is the male midwife is of interest for a number of reasons, some of which I have alluded to above. Setting aside his novelty value, he is included here more for the sake of presenting a complete picture of men in childbearing than the impact which his arrival has exerted on midwifery in the United Kingdom.

The reasons for men's move into midwifery, though well documented, remain obscure. The initial impetus occurred in the late 1960s and early 1970s (Lewis, 1991). This was the time when men, as part of the counter-culture, were beginning to stay with their partners during labour in hospital. It may be, as reported by one male midwife, that that shared experience had the effect of 'inspiring' a career change (Moore, 2000). The immediate, if questionably relevant, reaction was one of general opposition from nursing and medical organisations. In addition, and probably more significantly, opposition was voiced by the two royal colleges most closely involved, namely the Royal College of Midwives and the Royal College of Obstetricians and Gynaecologists. The reasons for such surprisingly united antagonism were said to relate to the nature of the occupational group, the likelihood of women's opposition and the labour force, that is resource, implications of the necessary large-scale chaperoning which was anticipated.

The source from which antagonism was not forthcoming was Harold Wilson's Labour government, which, in 1975, was in the process of manoeuvring the sex discrimination legislation on to the statute book. Special arrangements were introduced for midwives when this legislation was enacted. The Sex Discrimination Act dispensed with the legal ban on men practising as midwives which had applied since 1926 (Donnison, 1973). In place of this ban, transitional arrangements which restricted the entry of men into midwifery came into force.

Two experimental midwifery courses were drawn up on to which men would be accepted. One was offered in England and the other in Scotland. These courses were evaluated and the anxieties which had fuelled the opposition to the male midwife were shown to be unfounded (Speak and

Aitken-Swan, 1982). Probably more importantly, these courses established that the numbers of men seeking to become midwives was not large. Thus anxieties about rapid and fundamental changes in the nature of the midwifery profession resulting from male midwives' presence proved similarly groundless.

Lewis attempts to be reassuring that a phenomenon which has become established in nursing will not develop in midwifery. This phenomenon comprises the small minority of male practitioners occupying a large proportion of the most senior posts (1991: 298). It may be, though, that such a reassuring conclusion is somewhat premature.

The entrance of the father on to the scene

As mentioned above, the entrance of the father in to the birthing arena is a late twentieth-century development. The father's negotiation of his entrance is not well documented, so I attempt here to outline the sequence of events. The most valuable account of this development is the one written by Woollett and colleagues (1982). These authors initially regret the lack of data and then go on to draw on baby and child care manuals to trace the father's progress. These sources originally regarded the father as more than likely to provoke fear and anxiety in the woman, and thus he was considered to be 'a serious menace' (Dick-Read, 1942). This guarded view of the father's contribution continued to be endorsed by Spock (1979), who saw the father in traditional terms. This role comprised transporting the woman to the maternity unit and then, possibly, pacing the waiting room or, more likely, drinking in a bar. Woollett and colleagues credit Kitzinger (1972) with being the first childbirth guru to recognise the father as having a real role.

The changing rhetoric has been outlined in numerical terms. The gradual increase in the number of fathers attending the birth is shown by data from Nottingham (Lewis, 1986: 61). In 1960 fathers attended 8 per cent of births, but by 1980 84 per cent were present during labour with 67 per cent of fathers staying for the birth. Woollett and colleagues (1982: 73) report similar figures in more affluent areas of England, but without details of whether the father stayed for the actual birth.

There appears to have been some variation in the acceptance of the father and, similarly, in how continuously he was permitted to be present. In a study which involved data collection in England in 1984, Garcia and Garforth found some variability (1989). Only 40 per cent of units (n = 88) stated that the father was never excluded, while in 22 per cent of units (n = 48) the father could be excluded at the 'doctor's discretion' (1989: 157). Macfarlane also found that the father's route into the labour room was less than straightforward (1977). In an unnamed maternity unit the father was making good progress, but, as Garcia and Garforth found, this unit did not permit the father into the operating theatre. Macfarlane suggests that this maternity unit had changed its policy so that, in order to exclude him, assisted births happened in the operating theatre rather than in the labour room (1977: 58). Thus the father was not allowed to be present and his progress was again blocked.

Apart from anecdotal accounts (Beech and Thomas, 2001), the father's presence in the labour room does not seem to have been recorded in the literature before 1974 (RCM, 1995a). I have, however, a vivid recollection of the interest aroused among the labour ward staff at a maternity unit in 1968 that a father should choose to stay for the duration of his partner's prolonged and highly medicalised labour. The father further impressed the staff by sketching a cartoon showing his partner in labour; in it she was represented as an octopus with the tentacles replaced by tubes, catheters, wires, drains and other impedimenta.

The opposition to the father's presence in labour was argued in terms of preventing infection, avoiding nuisances, such as fathers fainting, or as the father being perverted (Cronenwett and Newmark, 1974; Richman, 1982: 93). A midwife argued that birth, as a 'nursing procedure', should not be witnessed by relatives (Dixon, 1977). Refusing to 'compromise with the public', she stated that birth is too 'dangerous' for the father to be involved. Dixon's clearly outdated views met a torrent of invariably hostile responses. Many of the correspondents reported encouraging the father's presence and having done so for as long as twenty years. These respondents cited a family orientation, nature, support, companionship, personal experience and the woman's wishes as reasons *for* the father to be present (Correspondence, 1977: 9–11).

Alongside Dixon's letter, a father recounted his personal experience of seeking to be with his wife for the birth of their second child, having been surprised at how right it was for him to be present at their first child's birth (Backwell, 1977). The woman was being subjected to a routinely medicalised induction and birth. During the labour, which deteriorated into a confrontation, the staff became increasingly defensive and communication appears to have been abysmal. Whereas the father was initially excluded, he was eventually admitted for the birth and given challenging tasks for which he was quite unprepared, such as administering 'gas and air' (1977: 271). Backwell points up other inconsistencies in his experience, such as, first, the paradoxical attitudes of antenatal and labour personnel regarding his presence. The second major inconsistency is the 'prudishness' of the staff in relation to bedpans, shaving and vaginal examinations, but not the actual birth. An even more disconcerting aspect of this personal account is that the couple's complaints to the Health Services Commissioner (Ombudsman) were not all upheld. Further, those complaints that were upheld failed to be operationalised by the Health Authority.

It is apparent from Backwell's account and from my observation in 1968 that the father was gradually being accepted into the labour room at a time when maternity care was undergoing its own 'revolution'. Thus, the father was being allowed in to witness what was developing into a maelstrom of changing practices and changing roles. In the next chapter there is an opportunity to examine closely two of these changing roles and, in subsequent chapters, their implications for men and the process of childbirth.

Conclusion

On the basis of this brief examination of the relevant historical and cross-cultural literature, certain themes are clearly emerging which provide useful insights into the background of the man's input into childbearing. The literature shows that the man's participation in childbearing, either as an attendant or as a partner, is not usual. Further, in those societies where he does participate, his arrival, in terms of the history of the human race, is relatively recent.

The cross-cultural literature shows the widespread tendency of men to avoid childbearing situations. In order to compensate for his inability to contribute directly, certain behaviours have become standard, which to some extent help him to find a role. In spite of their avoidance, even though the man is not prepared to be physically present, he and others have developed an elaborate system of prohibitions which serve to control the woman and her attendants around the time of the birth. Thus, in a multitude of cultures, the man is able to enforce the usual societal balance of power by indirect means. Obviously there may be benefits for the childbearing woman and her attendants in following these rituals. Not least among these is the maintenance of a well-ordered, if male-dominated, society.

In historical terms, the disruption of this status quo has occurred with the development of a new medical intervention or when the culture has been undergoing some major form of transition. Such transitions are those which have constituted a serious threat to the stability of the society and the culture or cultures which it comprises.

Thus it is apparent that the indirect control of childbearing by men may be a 'steady state'. In certain periods of social upheaval, opportunities have arisen and been grasped by men to gain control over this 'women's business' (Donnison, 1973; Mander and Reid, 2002). In this way the existing balance of power in the birthing room has been overturned by men being able to exert their power directly over a relatively compliant female population.

Chapter 2

The midwife and medical men

Introduction

In this chapter I redeploy the concepts which I introduced in Chapter 1 to provide a foundation for an examination of the role of one particular group of men in the childbearing scenario. In the last chapter I established the gendered nature of both the historical and the cross-cultural backgrounds of maternity care. I now proceed to consider the evidence relating to the current Western European situation. This leads inevitably to a contemplation of the implications of any gender imbalance in care provision for both the provider and, indirectly, for the consumer of maternity care.

The emphasis on medical *men* in the title of this chapter may benefit from being explained, or even justified. The domination of men in medicine may be criticised as being a purely historical artefact without any modern relevance. Evidence to support this criticism may be found in the data produced on university medical school entrants. These data show that, even in a traditional university, a majority of those embarking on a medical education at the time of writing are female (Edinburgh University, 2002). Further data to support this criticism come from the publications of feminists working in the sociology of the professions, for example, Lorber (1993, 1997).

The fallacious nature of this criticism, though, becomes apparent in a more detailed examination of, for example, Lorber's work (1997: 66). She draws on research evidence to show that the stereotypically 'womanly' characteristics, such as warmth, empathy and ability to listen and communicate, are not highly valued among medical practitioners. For this reason, as well as others relating to women's discontinuous career patterns, women who display these stereotypical characteristics, and women in general, are unlikely to find themselves in the most senior positions in the medical hierarchy. It may be further suggested, on the basis of personal observation, that some women medical practitioners may overcompensate for their lack of a male gender. This means that, in the interests of their professional advancement, they may check their womanliness and emphasise their stereotypically masculine characteristics (Stephens, 1998: 452). Oakley pursues this argument through to its logical conclusion, by demonstrating that misogyny is particularly rife among obstetricians and gynaecologists (1984: 254). In this chapter, however, the only assumption being made is that the medical power base, at least in the maternity field, is inherently masculine.

This balance or imbalance of power, as the title of this chapter suggests, carries implications for both the midwife and the medical man. A fundamental aspect of our understanding of the relationship between these two occupational groups is the terminology which we use to describe them. The dictionary definition of the word 'midwife' is rather narrow in its interpretation of midwifery practice: 'a woman who assists others in childbirth' (Macdonald, 1981: 829). The dictionary, however, does go on to explain this word's Old English origins: 'O.E>. *mid*, with (Ger. Mit/Gr. meta), *wif*, woman'. What may be less well known is that the obstetrician, namely the medical person who is 'qualified to practice obstetrics', derives his name from the Latin: 'ob, before, *stare*, to stand' (Macdonald, 1981: 909).

Thus it is apparent that the two occupational groups' names are diametrically opposed in their origins. This opposition is further characterised by the way that the terms define a totally different relationship with the woman client. The difference in relationship is represented both in terms of the attendant's alignment with the woman and the attendant's posture. It may also be appropriate to consider the possibility of the implications of the names' origins, i.e. Old English versus Latin. These origins may reflect the holders' attitude to their activities and their occupational aspirations.

Situating the contenders

In order to examine the relationship between the midwife and her medical colleagues, I use the framework introduced by the sociologist of maternity care, Raymond DeVries, in his critical analysis of the international status of the midwife (1996). He categorised into three major groups the factors which influence the status of the midwife. In this way he provided a comprehensive outline of the most contentious interprofessional issues in childbearing. I consider that the same groups of factors may be used appropriately to explore the relationship between the provider of midwifery care and her medical colleagues.

Technologies and techniques

In this section I take the liberty of interpreting DeVries' term 'technology' rather more loosely than he does; thus this term encompasses a wide range of hardware, techniques and other innovations which have been introduced into the childbearing arena. In the same way as the midwifery (later obstetric) forceps were smuggled into the birthing room in an oversized chest to disguise their true nature (Chapter 1, p. 29; see also Wilson, 1995: 53), other innovations have also been brought in surreptitiously. In this clandestine process, the 'cover' which was used is likely to have been that the innovation was intended to help a small and well-defined group of women. Following this progress, though, the 'benefits' to this small group of women have been deemed too great to be denied to the large majority of women. On the basis of this rationale the majority of women have become 'routinely' subjected to the innovative intervention. Thus, the 'technological imperative' is clearly seen to be operating. The example mentioned above, namely the 'midwifery' forceps, was invented originally by the Chamberlen family. These instruments were intended to avoid the necessity of 'destructive operations' on a probably dead fetus, in order to save the life of the moribund mother (see Chapter 1, p. 29). Their use, however, spread to become routine. In this way the analogy is continued, to the extent of the abominable North American intervention known as the 'prophylactic forceps operation' (DeLee, 1920). It may be that this sequence of events has happened too frequently to be worthy of comment. I suggest, however, that rehearsing some examples is appropriate here to demonstrate the more immediate issues.

To continue the analogy with the 'midwifery' forceps, Arney (1982: 26) indicates that this invention was intended to secure the Chamberlens' income rather than to reduce women's suffering, or to extend human well-being or knowledge. That their innovation was destined to bring about fundamental changes to human childbearing by converting it from a domestic experience to a pseudo-scientific specialty was probably unknown and unknowable by the Chamberlens. In this section the long-term implications and repercussions of some other selected examples of innovative birth interventions are examined.

Routine obstetric ultrasound

In the same way as the story of the introduction of the 'midwifery' forceps makes for gripping reading, so too does the invention of ultrasound (Oakley, 1984). A truly swashbuckling character of the old school, obstetrician Ian Donald drew on his Second World War experience in the RAF to realise the potential for radar and sonar to be used to 'detect flaws in women' (TVS, 2002; Willocks, 1996). The development of obstetric ultrasound was slow and discouraging until, the story goes, Donald was presented with the opportunity to correct the grave misdiagnosis of an ovarian cyst. Writing in 1968, Donald admitted that all he needed was an 'inexhaustible supply of living patients with fascinating clinical problems . . . to get ahead really fast' (Willocks, 1996). Obviously at that time the 'supply' was not as plentiful as might have been wished. It is my personal recollection that at that time in the maternity unit where Donald practised, only two or three pregnant women per day were being investigated using ultrasound. This was probably just as well, as the pregnant women were far from enthralled at having to drink one litre of fluid to ensure a sufficiently full bladder and *then* to await the arrival of the obstetrician. The use of warmed olive oil as the contact medium was a minor compensation. Obviously, at that time ultrasound was being used highly selectively. Since then this situation has changed out of all recognition, to the extent that ultrasound examinations in early pregnancy, and possibly later too, have become effectively routine. It is the routinisation of this investigation which has raised a number of issues.

Perhaps the only incontrovertible fact in this scenario is that women generally appreciate having their 'scan'. It is possible that Green and colleagues found how much women like ultrasound when they referred to the scan as the 'high spot' of the woman's antenatal care (1992: 75). These researchers identified, however, that women have little perception that the scan could possibly be anything other than a chance to 'meet' their baby. Even less did the women contemplate that there might actually be a 'down side' to this first encounter (see below).

A major benefit of routine ultrasound is the improved gestational assessment which it provides. This has been measured in terms of the reduction in the number of inductions of labour for postmaturity (Neilson, 2002). This benefit may indeed be a case of 'being damned with faint praise', when the major effect is to reduce the incidence of potentially iatrogenic medical intervention. A finding that may surprise even enthusiasts, however, is the absence of any effect of routine ultrasound on the perinatal mortality rate. This failure to reduce perinatal deaths leads to the crucial question of whether the huge capital financial and staff costs of routine ultrasound are the most effective way of using these finite health resources.

The crucial question of the safety of routine ultrasound has not yet been satisfactorily answered (Beech and Robinson, 1996). Even Neilson's systematic review is not able to be more than lukewarm in defence of routine ultrasound:

> the benefit of the demonstrated advantages would need to be considered against the theoretical possibility that the use of ultrasound during pregnancy could be hazardous, and the need for additional resources. At present, there is no clear evidence that ultrasound examination during pregnancy is harmful.
>
> (Neilson, 2002)

This cautious twenty-first-century recommendation should be contrasted with ultrasound's early advocates. Among them were Campbell and Little, who expounded as early as 1980 that ultrasound: 'should be regarded as an integral part of prenatal care' (1980: 27).

Because of the effortlessness of the acceptance of ultrasound into maternity care, if for no other reason, its introduction is important. It represents a prime example of the ease with which a quite unevaluated technology is able to gain enthusiastic recognition and promotion among the medical fraternity.

The crucial significance of routine ultrasound, however, may be found in two important areas. The first is the diametrically opposed yet rarely articulated aims of the two participants in this scenario. As mentioned above, the woman's agenda is that she wishes both to 'meet' her baby and to be assured that all is well with the child. The medical practitioner, on the other hand, is working to a totally different agenda. He is searching for fetal abnormalities which will constitute reasons to intervene in the pregnancy; that is, by terminating it (Reid, 1990). These fundamental yet paradoxical aims of routine ultrasound constitute a fertile area for disappointment. As Bricker and colleagues observe: 'Such features may augment the potential for anxiety, shock and disappointment when the scan shows a problem' (2000).

The second main area which has been affected by the introduction of routine ultrasound is the change in the status of the woman's knowledge of her pregnancy. Prior to the advent of routine ultrasound the woman, through her body and her feelings, held all information regarding the well-being of the fetus. Information on the date and nature of her last menstrual period, when she first feels fetal movements (the quickening date) and the vigour and continuation of the fetal movements, were sought of the woman as a matter of course. Thus the woman occupied a privileged status in relation to her baby. She was *responsible* for knowing her baby and, thus, for the child's welfare. Routine ultrasound has effectively downgraded her and her unique knowledge. Her role as her baby's guardian has been bypassed, demoting her to little more than an observer of these developments. She is no longer uniquely responsible for being aware of her pregnancy, as her knowledge has been superseded by technical equipment. In the same way as the fetus is no longer in a unique position as 'the lord at the end of the cord', the mother is no longer privileged to share that singular relationship. This ability to subject the woman and the fetus to comprehensive observation, with the obvious implications for intervention, has been compared to the concept of a 'panopticon' which comprises an all-seeing, all-controlling and all-powerful machine (Arney, 1982: 30).

Routine continuous electronic fetal monitoring in labour

It is appropriate that I should consider routine continuous electronic fetal monitoring (CEFM) next to ultrasound because of the close relation of the technology. CEFM uses ultrasound to record the fetal heart rate (FHR) unless a scalp electrode is used, as is currently happening less frequently due to risks of HIV. The rationale for observing the fetal heart rate is that it is assumed to correlate with the oxygenation of the fetus and, most importantly, the fetal brain. Thus the FHR is deemed to carry some prognostic value. These observations may be made using the Pinards (monaural) stethoscope or continuous or intermittent electronic methods. Because of the similarities in technology, CEFM came to be widely used at approximately the same time as ultrasound. However, that it is used mainly during labour and that it does not have the 'happy' associations of ultrasound, means that the issues are somewhat different.

For the woman in labour, the usual methods of CEFM carry a number of implications. Some women find the transducers, and the belts used to hold them in position, uncomfortable. Further, the high sensitivity of the transducers may mean that their optimal functioning demands some limitation of the woman's mobility. For this reason, she is likely to be discouraged from moving about, at a time when adopting different positions would help to alleviate her pain.

Intermittent auscultation (IA) using either a Pinard's stethoscope or a handheld ultrasound device usually involves the midwife 'listening in' at least once every 15 minutes when the woman is in established labour. Clearly, this highly labour-intensive method of observation is likely to prevent one midwife from caring for more than one labouring woman. This staff allocation may not be considered to be the most cost-effective use of limited resources. Experienced midwives have told me that, when they are required to care for more than one woman, they prefer that the mother be monitored continuously rather than have no FHR observations. Kargar (1990) takes this argument a stage further when she suggests that CEF monitors may be used to actually substitute for midwifery staff, and thus, reduce the midwifery salary costs. This staffing 'benefit' of CEFM is also argued from a North American perspective by Simkin, who states: '[the attendant] can leave the bedside more easily to take care of other women, do other chores or take a break' (1986: 20). In spite of these supposed 'benefits' CEFM may actually cause the midwife more work in terms of frequently explaining to the parents what the monitor is or is not doing, reporting possibly falsely suspicious traces to medical personnel, and undertaking the multiplicity of interventions necessary following a questionable trace.

The midwife's unique skills may be used differently in the context of CEFM. Simkin, writing in North America, suggests that reading a printout may be more intellectually stimulating for the midwife than 'listening in' using a Pinard's stethoscope (1986). This suggestion is surprising in view of the difficulty which I have found some personnel experience in using a Pinard's.

Although the reading and interpretation of the trace (or 'strip') may be presented as an exact science, there is evidence that this is far from the case (Zain et al., 1998). Hypothetical traces presented to differing grades and disciplines of staff on different occasions have shown both inter- as well as intra-observer reliability to be low. Staff education has been used in attempts to resolve such difficulties (Beckmann et al., 1997).

In the current climate of defensive obstetrics it may be an advantage that the printed trace is a permanent record of the fetal condition. This may be perceived to constitute a defence in the event of a poor perinatal outcome, such as the demise of the baby, and litigation. In their reply to this perception, however, Capstick and Edwards' legal opinion is that these traces are, at best, a mixed blessing and may well be 'a sword turned against the doctor' (1991: 823). These legal experts recommend certain precautions which practitioners should take to protect themselves from CEFM-related litigation; such as limiting its use to situations of established value and recording any 'wait and see' decisions. In support of this view, Keirse provides a hilarious rebuttal of the defensive use of CEFM. He argues that any court which accepts a trace as evidence is being seriously misled by 'wise men and women' (1986: 256). The brunt of his paper relates to the way in which courts are expected to accept this 'evidence' as a defence, when the real evidence (from randomised controlled trials) is equivocal to say the least.

The main issue which arises out of the use of CEFM relates to the acquisition and use of knowledge in medical practice. The problem which underlies this issue is the faith of medical men in the assumption that any pathophysiology is invariably identifiable by technology. This assumption ignores, first, the limitations of the essentially human interpretation of the traces and, second, the data presented by the nine high-quality randomised controlled trials (Thacker et al., 2002). These trials show the limited value of CEFM. The only clearly significant benefit appears to be that neonatal convulsions are reduced by the use of routine CEFM in labour. This is not a justification of routine CEFM, since such convulsions have no serious long-term effects. Further, Thacker and colleagues emphasise the increase in interventive births – such as caesarean – due to CEFM, which has implications for the woman, the baby and the maternity service.

This examination of CEFM points up the inability of the medical practitioner to accept research findings which are clearly contrary to his own underlying belief system. This system of beliefs may constitute a theoretical framework, in which he has been educated and in which he may have practised for all of his working life. This leads inevitably to the question of whether medical men are as truly 'scientific' in their approach to care as they claim. This question will be explored further as this chapter progresses.

Other technologies

These two examples of childbearing technologies (ultrasound and CEFM) have indicated a number of issues which impinge on the relationship between the midwife and medical men. To this short list could be added any number of other examples which would demonstrate similar issues such as the Heyns bag, laminaria tents, the Cardiff infusion system, routine magnesium trisilicate administration, routine stilboestrol administration, the Elliott bed, the Iowa trumpet and the Drew-Smythe catheter. Thus, although the nature and extent of the technology varies hugely, the issues still persist. The problems relating to a form of technology which is barely deserving of the name have been highlighted by Murphy-Black (1990). She reminisces about all the pubic shaves which have been inflicted on women, causing each woman to leave the maternity hospital with 'a baby and an itch'. These outcomes are attributed to the invention of the safety razor in the 1920s. She regrets that it took sixty years for research to show that the application of this technology did more harm than good and even longer for the research to be accepted by the medical decision-makers. In conclusion, Murphy-Black questions rightly how long it will take for the widely recognised research on CEFM to be translated into practice.

Fetal focus

It should not be surprising that technology's increasing ability to study the fetus has apparently altered the focus of care in childbearing (Weaver, 2002: 232). While the fetus had long been unknown and unknowable, the woman's welfare was the only real concern of her attendants. With the possibility of listening to, visualising, taking specimens from and operating on the fetus, a more 'fetocentric' form of maternity care has evolved. This new state is depicted by Wagner in the slightly surprising terms of the physicians being the 'defenders of the rights of the unborn or the just born' (1994: 31). As mentioned above, this development may have served to transform the woman into an observer, rather than the leading actor in the drama which is childbirth. This effect has been aggravated by the increasingly reductionist approach to childbirth in which the components of the woman's childbearing experience are artificially separated (Fleming, 2002). Probably more significantly, care is provided by different personnel depending on the stage of childbearing and whether the woman or her baby is affected. Thus, the concept of 'fetocentrism' may have contributed to the discontinuous nature of modern maternity care.

Unfortunately, though, the problems of the 'fetocentric' approach may not relate only to the satisfaction or otherwise of the childbearing woman. Drawing on the work of Foucault, Williams (1997) shows the escalating nature of knowledge subsequent to technological developments. Knowledge, in turn, provides a firmer base for increasing power and the two 'operate in a mutually generative fashion' (1997: 236). In this way, she argues, the medical control over childbearing which was strengthened with the establishment of antenatal care in the early days of the twentieth century (Oakley, 1982) is legitimated further. This control is unlikely to benefit the other actors in the childbearing scene. Williams gives the historical example of routine X-rays in pregnancy and the current practice of chorionic villus sampling; many others may be added to her short list, including those mentioned above.

The broad approach

These technologies should in no way be viewed as discreet entities. Their introduction has been part and parcel of the changes which have been termed the 'Childbirth Revolution'. Crucially, these changes have affected the healthy woman enjoying an uncomplicated experience of childbearing as well as the midwife who provides her care. Thus, the woman is likely to be subjected to interventions which are 'technological', but which also have more immediate bodily effects. Examples of such routines would include the use of episiotomy (Graham, 1997), augmentation or acceleration of the first stage of labour (O'Driscoll *et al.*, 1993) and active management of the third stage (Prendiville *et al.*, 2002). The research evidence base of each of these procedures has been questioned and their use not supported, but their widespread implementation as routine practices persists. For the individual woman each procedure has affected her experience of childbearing. Collectively, however, they have diminished the role of the midwife and correspondingly enhanced the obstetrician's status.

CASCADE OF INTERVENTION

An excellent example of this combination of effects may be found in the phenomenon which has become known as the 'cascade of intervention' (Mold and Stein, 1986; Varney Burst, 1983). Goer (1995: 332) regards the cascade as beginning with the woman being confined to bed for the purpose of routine CEFM. Such immobilisation is likely to slow uterine contractions. In order to counteract this 'dytocia', an oxytocic is likely to be administered intravenously. These drugs are, anecdotally, said to increase the severity of pain, for which epidural analgesia would be provided. The slow progress clearly associated with epidural analgesia, with or without incomplete rotation of the fetal head and fetal hypoxia, would constitute an indication for either an assisted or an operative birth (Mander, 1993).

The origins of the 'cascade of intervention' are recognised by Mold and Stein (1986). These two medical practitioners admit the imperative for the obstetrician to be seen to be doing *something* during uncomplicated labour. His activity is not only for the benefit of the childbearing woman, but it also serves to diminish his own anxiety about a process over which he realises he has little or no control. This is a stereotypically masculine reaction, to which I will be making further reference (see Chapter 4).

The self-fulfilling nature of the expectations inherent in the cascade of intervention relate to the 'as if' rule (Oakley, 1989: 219). She argues that by treating all childbearing women as if problems are about to develop, the problems *do* actually materialise. In this way the existence of the cascade is perpetuated in the form of a self-fulfilling prophecy. In a similar vein, but even more contentiously, Goer (1995) argues that medical personnel have insufficient insight into the cascade of intervention to recognise that it is predominantly of their own making.

THE PARTOGRAM

A deceptively simple form of technology which may be related to the cascade of intervention is the partogram or partograph (formerly the cervicograph (Philpott, 1972)). This is a paper document which records 'intrapartum details in a pictorial manner, enabling rapid identification of abnormal labour patterns' (Lavender et al., 1999). This definition is problematical for two reasons. First, it assumes that a normal pattern of labour exists and that its nature is known. This may not be the case, since even uncomplicated labour is highly individual and may be affected by phenomena which are as intangible as the woman's current state of mind. Second, the definition omits to mention the automatic corollary of identifying an abnormal labour pattern. Inevitably, once identified, any abnormal pattern would need to be returned to normal by the use of intravenous oxytocic drugs. The crucial section of the partogram is the line in which the state of the cervix or, more precisely, the dilation of the cervix is recorded (IPPF, 2002). In the partogram recommended by the WHO an 'alert' line and an 'action' line are provided in case the rate of cervical dilation does not reach the required speed.

The concept of the partogram deserves to be criticised on the grounds that it is unsound; it assumes incorrectly that the speed and continuity of progress in labour is common to all women and that it is predictable. The individuality of each woman and her labour should be recognised and not be prescribed according to some notional standard. The partogram assumed its current significance due to its association with active management of labour. This aggressive form of labour intervention is claimed to have been introduced originally to prevent women from having to suffer the trauma of prolonged labour (O'Driscoll et al., 1993). The partogram's widespread use is based on research which is less than convincing to the point of being seriously flawed (Rosser, 1994). The question which has still to be asked is whether the partogram has been introduced for the benefit of the labouring woman or for the convenience of her medical attendants.

PLACE OF BIRTH

The admission of a woman to hospital for childbirth is not usually regarded as constituting a technology per se. Being in a hospital environment, though, certainly increases the likelihood that she will be exposed to a wide range of technological interventions. Clearly these technologies, which carry iatrogenic potential, would not be available to her and her attendants if she were in her own home (Olsen and Jewell, 2002). Writing about the history of childbearing, Cahill endorses this view when she reflects on the inaccuracy of the lay view of hospitalisation when she states: 'women largely assume that hospital means [medical] experts and that surely means a safer birth' (2001: 340).

The home birth debate has for far too long foundered on the issue of safety. This medical confounding tactic has passed widely unrecognised, in spite of the lack of attention given to the dubious safety of the institutional form of birth. The confusion has been compounded by the lack of differentiation between planned from unplanned home births. These two birth experiences share so little in common that it is a constant surprise that they continue to bear the same name.

The removal of birth from home to hospital was fuelled by a series of government reports which culminated in the infamous Peel Report (DHSS, 1970). As well as a pivotal role being played by the general practitioner in maternity care, this document recommended that 100 per cent of births should happen in hospital. In the presence of a declining birth rate and an increasing maternity bed provision, the medical establishment sought, through this report, to entrench its power base (Campbell, 1997). The Peel Report did this by recommending that all mothers should be able to 'benefit from the facilities available in hospital'. Peel's long-term implications are summarised by Sargent who maintains that this report 'confirmed the spurious desirability of hospitalised obstetric management of labour within a framework designed to limit choice for women' (2002: 42).

Following Peel, however, the data collected by Tew and the medical students she taught were originally intended to shore up the medical orthodoxy. The students' findings, however, proved to be heretical. The conclusions were subsequently rendered even more threatening to the medical establishment when, in response to her critics, Tew exposed the massive discrepancy in outcomes between planned and unplanned home births (Tew, 1984).

Since this original work, other authorities have used this scenario to demonstrate the medical fraternity's disconcertingly shaky scientific foundations. As Campbell and MacFarlane have scathingly observed: 'Perhaps the most striking feature of the debate . . . is the way that policy has been formed with very little reference to the evidence' (1987).

A systematic review of the meagre evidence on the place of birth has been undertaken by Olsen and Jewell (2002). These researchers confidently conclude that neither hospital birth nor planned home birth has been shown to be any safer or less safe for the low-risk woman. On the basis of this conclusion they recommend that women should be encouraged to plan a home birth rather than plan to give birth in hospital.

Another important issue, which will re-emerge later and which also resonates with the concept of the 'cascade of intervention' (see p. 44 above), is raised by a vocal and articulate consumer representative. Thomas (2002) highlights a danger of institutional birth which serves to epitomise the 'prudence' underpinning much medical practice. She refers to 'the "just-in-case" routines' to which the woman may be subjected if she finds herself in labour somewhere other than 'on her own territory' (Thomas, 2002: 28). These ideas resonate with those of Oakley (1989: 219) mentioned above (p. 44). Such routines are clearly the first rivulets which eventually become the cascade.

In her Finnish work studying the meaning of home birth, Viisainen (2001) makes reference to the ideas of Davis-Floyd. Viisainen discusses the powerful control which biomedical knowledge exerts over many aspects of human life. She regards obstetrical intervention in childbearing as an example of such control. Drawing heavily on North American sources, she espouses an 'alternative childbirth ideology', which comprises a coalition of women and midwives to alter the experience of both groups. Viisainen epitomises home birth as the ultimate example of resistance to the medical model, although she uses Davis-Floyd's terminology to rename it 'technocracy' (2001: 1110). The application of these ideas to the European context is more assumed than real, presumably on the basis that the more extreme North American example will be seen to inform the local picture.

This crucial significance of home birth also manifests itself in the work of Isherwood (2000/1). She writes in response to the UKCC's ill-fated foray into the uncharted wastes of the home birth debate (UKCC, 2001). In their ignorance, the UKCC made the unfortunate mistake of interpreting the home birth debate merely in terms of the resource issues raised by managers. Their resulting diktat comprised considerable heat with very little light. On the basis of this unhappy misunderstanding, Isherwood attempts to elucidate the meaning of home birth to mothers and to midwives. Her thoughts resonate profoundly with the findings of Viisainen's study. The resource argument barely deserves consideration, in view of the plethora of resource-hungry and unevaluated routines in maternity care. Isherwood points up the irrefutable significance of home birth to the midwife and medical practitioners. This means that home birth is a form of care in which no obstetrician would deign to involve himself. Thus, it becomes a defining characteristic of the midwife, in that it is something which she is both able and willing to offer. In this way, it may be suggested that home birth may be regarded as constituting a test of the midwifery profession's credentials. This concept of a test has been referred to as a 'shibboleth' and it is particularly appropriate in this context, since it was originally supposed to have been used to differentiate a friend from an enemy.

NON-CONSENSUAL CAESAREAN

The terms 'non-consensual', 'en/forced' and 'court-ordered' may be used synonymously to indicate a caesarean operation performed without the woman's fully informed consent. Often this lack of consent means that this operation is undertaken against her will. It is this form of intervention which highlights most clearly the potential for conflict between different sources of knowledge and action in the childbearing arena.

Following her study of court-ordered caesareans in the USA, Jordan (1997: 59) demonstrates the depth of self-knowledge used by women declining caesarean. Although assumptions and accusations of irrationality or mental incompetence may be made by medical personnel and lawyers, she found that this was far from the case. Beech cites a number of cases as examples, such as the 'poor' New York woman (1996: 1) whose main concern was her need to have an intact and healthy body in order to care for her nine older children. Jordan focuses on the gulf between the woman's knowledge of her own social situation, bodily functioning and value system and the medical knowledge-base. She goes on to show how certain 'knowledges' may become 'socially sanctioned, consequential, even official' (1997: 60). In this way decisions about surgical intervention in childbirth against the woman's will and without her involvement or knowledge have been legitimated. The disregard of other people's knowledge reflects a professional arrogance which should not surprise those acquainted with the health care arena. Even more disconcerting, though, is the phenomenon identified by Jordan, whereby women and others allow their own knowledge to be 'superseded and delegitimised' by medical personnel (1997: 61). In this way women's confidence, including midwives', is effectively undermined.

The knowledge-base used by medical practitioners to underpin such decisions is explored by Cahill (2001). She identifies that interventions, such as non-consensual caesarean, are not based on what Weaver terms 'value free, rational science' (2002: 239). They are based on stereotypically masculine assumptions about women, which have the twin effects of compromising and disempowering the women for whom care is being provided (Cahill, 2001: 340). The rationale for such a decision-making process is not only misogynistic, but is also associated with a form of obstetric personal insurance policy. This policy involves avoiding censure for not intervening in situations of uncertainty, such as uncomplicated labour. The corollary is that, should there be any less than favourable outcomes and the practitioner had not intervened, dire censure would be meted out by fellow professionals (Savage, 1998).

As well as the different knowledges operating and the medical compulsion to intervene, there appears to be another crucial player in this scenario. The role played by the lawyer is not insignificant, as argued by Hewson in her paper entitled 'Court-ordered caesarean: ethical triumph or surgical rape?' (1994: 1). The legal judgment to order a caesarean for the benefit of Mrs S' fetus was a landmark example of the all too cosy relationship between medical personnel and and their legal brothers. Mrs S was excluded from this relationship as she was excluded from all aspects of the decision that she should undergo a caesarean (Weaver, 2002: 234). The medico–legal dyad ignored the woman's knowledge, which was derived from her religious faith and previous experience of being threatened with an unnecessary caesarean. The legal process was used to enforce an entirely different kind of knowledge. This was the assumption made, first, by medical personnel on the basis of the value system outlined above. The second assumption was made by lawyers who had imported a fetocentric approach, which was alien to English law, from the USA (Weaver, 2002: 233).

In this way, what emerges from the non-consensual caesarean issue is the development of an alliance between lawyers and medical practitioners. Weaver, in recognising the existence of this cosy relationship (2002: 240), generously attributes it to the common socio-economic background shared by both groups. She further recognises the greater difficulty of being objective about the decision-making of a fellow professional than the decisions of a woman with a very different background. Irrespective of such rationalisation, the medico–legal alliance is united against the woman, as the non-consensual caesarean serves to deny to the woman the autonomy over her bodily integrity which is a fundamental requirement of ethical health care (Beauchamp and Childress, 1994).

Research and its use

Many of the examples cited in this section have supported Weaver's observation (2002: 239) that medicine's claims to be a 'value-free, rational science' do not withstand close scrutiny. I have given a number of examples, such as the research base being deficient, as in the case of the routine use of ultrasound in pregnancy. Whereas there is plentiful research demonstrating the limited benefits of routine CEFM, such research has been shown not to be well used in medical practice. The lack of research input into a plethora of other routine practices in maternity care has also been highlighted. In the case of the partogram, the quality of the research findings have been called into question. Occupationally endorsed value judgements, rather than research findings, have been shown to predominate in situations such as non-consensual caesarean. Similarly, unfounded medical prejudices have been shown to have influenced at least a generation of UK policy-makers in the context of home birth. Thus it is necessary to consider whether medicine's scientific credentials are more aspirational than real.

It is not, however, possible to deny that medicine has done a good job of effectively persuading the public and the policy-makers of these scientific credentials. That even midwives have been convinced of the quality of medical research emerged in a small study by Hicks (1992). She found that midwives were more negatively critical of a research paper which they perceived to be written by a midwife, than when they perceived the same paper to be written by a medical practitioner. Although Hicks attributed this tendency to a gender bias, the possibility of an occupational factor should not be ignored. When this tendency is converted into practice by midwife managers the outcome, as experienced by a midwife researcher, is even more disconcerting (Fleming, 2002: 73).

The medical approach to research has been examined in the context of one particular intervention in labour (Mander, 1994a). The occupational investment in epidural analgesia was not to be squandered for the sake of a lack of authoritative research. For this reason UK publications relating to the success or failure rates of this technique rely largely on anecdotal sources. The side effects for the woman have been minimised to the point of being ignored, with the benefits for the fetus being emphasised. Women's lack of knowledge and consumers' attitudes generally have been explored condescendingly. Such 'research' has served to do little more than alienate the representatives of consumer groups who question the use of such routine labour interventions. The abysmally low quality of the medical research into consumers' knowledge and attitudes leads to the conclusion that neither the research nor the knowledge and attitudes of consumers are of any great consequence to medical practitioners.

The general shortcomings of the positivist research methods, beloved of 'scientific' medical practitioners, are rehearsed by Oakley (1993: 215). She criticises the 'partial' view of reality which such methods inevitably permit when used by any dominant group; on the grounds that the less powerful group needs to understand not only itself but also the more powerful group. Thus she argues that the quantitative research methods are actually *less* scientific, since they provide an incomplete and distorted picture compared with the ways of knowing used by women. Oakley's argument focuses on the survey method of data collection, but her accusations of reductionism could be applied equally to the randomised controlled trial (RCT). She builds on this theme by identifying another weakness of quantitative research methods; this is their difficulty in coping with phenomena which are not easily measured or counted, such as intangibles like feelings and emotions. On this basis she recognises that the very existence of such phenomena may be ignored or denied due to their limited quantifiability. Thus it becomes apparent that medical research is largely irrelevant to childbearing issues, and when it is relevant there is likely to be a mismatch between methods and applications to practice.

The weaknesses of medical research would be of little significance were it not for research having been incorporated into government policy. The introduction of the concept of clinical governance (DoH, 1998) was disconcerting and not only because of the obscure terminology. This concept linked quality issues with research/audit and risk management. The research base, however, emphasises the importance of 'evidence', which ordinarily excludes the more stereotypically feminine research methods and sources of knowledge.

This traditional definition of evidence has been called into question by Wickham (2000: 149). She suggests that the usual medically oriented view needs to be transformed in the context of childbearing. This is partly due to the inappropriateness of much positivist research, but also because of the dearth of relevant research into childbearing matters. She argues that, in addition to the knowledge provided by RCTs and other research, such sources as the experiences, intuitions, common sense and bodily knowledge of both woman and midwife should be included as evidence.

Summary

This examination of the application of technology in childbearing has pointed up the limitations of medical research. In spite of Cochrane's unmercifully scathing criticism of obstetricians' poor use of research (1972), they have remained too arrogant to deign to use research effectively. This sin of omission has been compounded by the requirement that other occupational groups should demonstrate 'evidence-based practice' through the implementation of clinical governance.

The social structure

Introduction

The social relationships between the practitioners who work alongside each other in the maternity area may not easily be divorced from their historical origins. Here, I consider these origins briefly before examining a major stumbling-block to harmonious relationships. I then examine the research which has studied the reality of the midwife working alongside her medical colleagues.

Origins

The history of the relationship between the midwife and her medical colleagues is long and undistinguished. Of particular interest in terms of research and publications has been the complex events leading up to the passage of the first Midwives Act (1902), which applied to England and Wales (Donnison, 1988). The medical and political machinations prior to the passage of the Act have (probably appropriately) attracted more attention than have the activities of and implications for midwives. Witz (1992) examines the inter-occupational relations between various groups of medical personnel and midwives. She recounts the medical strategy of 'gendered demarcation' of midwives' practice by de-skilling them to care only for 'normal or natural' childbearing (1992: 112). Witz goes on to compare this medical strategy with the midwives' 'closure' of the handywoman's livelihood. Thus, while trained and *bona fide* midwives were being subsumed under more restrictive medical regulation they were, in turn, tightening the screws on their own occupational competitors (Leap and Hunter, 1993). The midwife, it appears, was seeking to compensate for the limitation of the more lucrative aspects of her practice by, effectively, moving downmarket to take over the practice of her even more vulnerable handywoman competitor. In this way the map of the 'segmentation' of the market in childbearing services was effectively redrawn (Witz, 1992: 116).

Although the certification of the midwife eventually presaged the obliteration of the working-class handywoman, there were also other associated developments. The man-midwife (see Chapter 1) was in the process of completing his transformation to a professional , that is an obstetrician. This process of transformation was partly, in the interests of securing his market, into a more respectable practitioner who would attract a wealthier clientele. Assuming control over his less organised competitor, the midwife, would assist this in no small way. An intermediate stage in the process of the professionalisation of obstetrics was the foundation of the British College of Obstetricians and Gynaecologists in September 1929. The professionalisation process was completed when the College was awarded its Royal Charter in 1947, having been granted its 'Royal' title in 1938 (RCOG, 2002).

A further body blow threatened midwives' remaining autonomy when, in 1948, the National Health Service (NHS) came into being (Harcombe, 1999: 78). The damage to midwives was inflicted partly by the escalation of the hospitalisation of birth, as home birth had long been the midwife's power-base. The move of childbearing, and hence midwifery, into hospitals generated a population of patients for medical practice and teaching. In this way medical power was inflated by this development. In addition, childbearing was moving into an established system of institutions. This meant that the midwife was required to accept the existing balance of power. So, rather than continuing as an autonomous practitioner, the midwife became part of the patriarchal system beloved of Nightingale. In this system the medical practitioner was the dominant 'father' figure and the nurse or midwife acted out the mothering role.

Normality

The social structure among those practising in the maternity area is inevitably influenced and may be determined by the working environment. For many midwives, due to the hospitalisation of birth, this is a maternity unit. Such an institution brings with it a range of attributes which may serve to benefit or harm those who are involved.

A problem which profoundly affects the social structure, and which has existed since the term was used in 1902 to distinguish medical from midwifery practice, is the meaning of the term 'normal'. While the concept of abnormality in relation to childbearing is relatively easy to define in terms of pathology, normality may be more elusive. This problem has become both more significant and more challenging since technology and interventions in childbearing have been allowed to become routinised. An extension of the 'normality' debate is that, while the term has been used to maintain the boundary between midwifery and medical practice, the 'policing' of that boundary has invariably been by the medical personnel (Witz, 1992).

For too long normal birth has been defined by medical personnel in terms of the births in which they have no interest. This applies to the births in which intervention cannot be justified or which do not require instrumental assistance. For this reason the assisted breech birth by any attendant, and even more by the midwife, is in danger of becoming a historical phenomenon. Thus defining normality in terms of 'naturalness' appears to be less than helpful. The equation of normal with natural is rendered even less acceptable by the memories of American 'natural childbirth', which referred to any vaginal birth that fell short of the full panoply of interventions, namely general anaesthesia and prophylactic forceps.

Normal birth has been defined in statistical terms to indicate the most frequently occurring, that is the median, or the average or mean (Gould, 2000). Unfortunately, these definitions say little about the woman's experience or the midwife's contribution and more about the environment in which her birth happens. Gould also offers healthy or physiological as synonyms for normal, but this term may be unsatisfactory because every birth should be maintained within the bounds of good health. A number of measurable parameters are offered on the basis of authoritative publications (Gould, 2000: 421), but these carry the likelihood of defining normal birth out of existence. It may be that the midwife has inadvertently 'painted herself into a corner' through her adherence to the mantra of 'normal birth', imposed as it was in 1902. The time may be overdue for the midwife to assert her will to ensure that the labour and birth are normal in the sense that the woman decides they should be.

Such a recommendation, though, ignores the usual patriarchal relationships inherent in maternity hospitals. These relationships derive more from Nightingale's aspirations for nurses than twenty-first-century working arrangements. An example of the misunderstandings inherent in this organisation of maternity care appears in the work of Fawdry (1994), who argues that the midwife should accept more of his obstetrical work. This medical writer appears to be advocating that the midwife should become part of the obstetric team, but he neglects to state the all too obvious discipline of the team leader. Fawdry misses the point that the main issue in interprofessional relationships is one of decision-making. This means that the midwife will be making the decision about whether and when to refer the woman to a medical colleague on her own responsibility, rather than according to medically determined protocols. In the context of Fawdry's ideas, the concept of 'normality' is clearly being used as a red herring.

Working relationships

In her old yet still relevant paper, Sheahan (1972) contemplated the working relationship between the nurse and the medical practitioner. Unlikely as it may at first sound, this paper is highly relevant to the working arrangements between the midwife and her medical colleagues. Sheahan describes two theoretical frameworks to which the (nurse) practitioner may adhere. The first is the 'technological' expert, who practises in close proximity to the medical protocols and guidelines and who finds satisfaction in the more technical aspects of her role. The second framework is what Sheahan terms the 'professional', by which she means the practitioner who values the human opportunities provided by her role. She goes on to argue that the practitioner has an important function as a role model for those for whom she provides care. She must set an example by choosing where her allegiances lie within the hierarchical health care system. The obvious implication is that these should be with her clients rather than machines, techniques or other disciplines. The relevance of these ideas to current midwifery practice is abundantly clear.

Research undertaken at widely spaced intervals has shown not only the nature of the working relationship between the midwife and her medical colleagues, but also how little that relationship has changed over time. A qualitative study by Walker (1976) demonstrated clearly the role of the midwife in the labour ward setting, particularly in maintaining congenial working relationships in the interests of the women. This was in spite of medical assumptions of overall responsibility for the woman's care. The medical staff interviewed were unable to distinguish between midwifery and obstetrics, except in hierarchical terms, as articulated by one of the medical staff: 'Their role [midwives] is to assist the obstetrician – they're an assistant really' (1976: 135). Kitzinger and colleagues (1993) investigated a novel form of medical staffing but still found that the midwives are regarded as: 'my juniors, my deputies' (1993: 158).

Both Walker and Kitzinger and their colleagues recognised the communicative or manipulative skills which the midwife needs to practice in order to persuade junior medical staff of their responsibilities. These skills, as identified by Walker, are fundamental to ensure the smooth running of the labour ward. Kitzinger and colleagues found that these skills must be practised surreptitiously: 'You just have to make them feel important and learn how to pull the right strings' (1993: 156). This phenomenon was labelled as 'hierarchy maintenance work'.

Even more recently a study on communication was undertaken within one labour ward setting by Brownlee and colleagues (1996). The functioning of the labour area was found to be perceived more negatively by the medical staff than by the midwives. Even more different were the perceptions of staffing levels, with each group asserting that there were too many of the other group and not enough of their own. The authors rather generously attribute such observations to: 'basic misunderstandings of each other's roles' (Brownlee *et al.*, 1996: 493). These misunderstandings were found to be associated with a problem which has been mentioned already, namely the meaning of 'normal' labour and birth. Medical personnel sought to control, limit or reduce the practice of the midwife. To this end a senior registrar suggested there should be: 'Better definition of what constitutes a midwife's case' (1996: 494).

Midwives, on the other hand, appear to be trying to entrench their position in order to hold on to what progress they have made in establishing a more complete role. One midwife suggested the working relationships could be improved by: 'Doctors listening more to midwives' opinions' (1996: 494). This research is presented in an upbeat style with a distinctly positive spin. It does, however, clearly show the continuing anxieties of junior medical staff and the aspirations of more senior medical staff to more firmly control their midwife colleagues.

The medical version of the Brownlee *et al.* paper (Wallace *et al.*, 1995) is broadly similar, but raises certain important issues. The first major difference is this paper's greater methodological detail, which raises ethical issues relating to the data being collected 'without the knowledge of the medical or labour ward midwifery staff' (1995: 165). Second, the recommendation is made that the hierarchical 'training grade' structure of medicine should also be imposed on midwifery (1995: 169). Third, the authors seek to use their findings to criticise the development of birthing centres free of medical input (1995: 168). Once more the spin doctors' positive words have a hollow ring.

The culture

Organisation

As has been mentioned above in the context of the implications of the creation of the NHS for home birth (see p. 52), organisational changes have the potential to affect many aspects of a service. It is well recognised by systems theorists that many of these effects will operate out of range of the original change and will only be attributable to it with difficulty. One of the reasons for this is the complexity of organisations such as the NHS; Harrison and colleagues regard this as being due to the 'multiple and conflicting objectives and interests' among those who make up such an organisation (1992: 3). One of those interests emerges in Halford's analysis of institutions, in which the NHS emerges as a prime example of a gendered institution, with its gendered nature being a crucial characteristic (1997: 14). She emphasises that gender is in no way an optional extra or some form of add-on, but that this characteristic is intrinsic to the composition of this organisation. In further support of its gendered nature, Stephens details the features of the NHS which justify her description of it as demonstrating 'public patriarchy' (1998: 451). The most obvious manifestation of patriarchy is probably found in the male/female employment ratio, which results in a small number of powerful and highly valued men occupying the most influential and lucrative positions. The majority of the workforce, however, is female and undertakes relatively poorly paid, undervalued, caring work. Stephens' comparison of the NHS structure with a pyramid, with the women occupying the base, is appropriate.

Power and medical power

Power is a key concept in the culture of health care, operating as it does in a number of different ways and at a number of different levels. Power is exercised as means of influencing an outcome, and it materialises when the threat of some form of sanction is made (Harrison *et al.*, 1992). The threat may be more or less explicit, but its perception is the crucial factor. Inevitably the imbalance in the relationship is absolute; the exertion of power by one agent engenders dependence in the other, so that the relationship may be said to correlate inversely. The preceding stages involve the existence of conflict, which is resolved by compliance on one side, resulting in their dependence on the more powerful agent.

As many would-be reformers of the NHS have learned to their cost, medical power is one of its predominant characteristics. Thus, Harrison and colleagues reflect with feeling on the power of medical practitioners to resist challenges to 'their traditional ways of doing things' (1992: 2). Obviously, medical power does not only operate in the form of what these writers call 'macropower' (1992: 17), when it is large-scale policies that are affected. Macropower originated with the nineteenth-century agreement that the medical profession would be granted monopoly professional status in return for keeping its own house in order.

At least as significant as macropower in the present context is medical power in the form of 'micropower', which is exerted during individual encounters. This latter manifestation of power is likely to be reinforced by the dependence, or other subservient behaviour, on the part of the other individual. Such behaviour may manifest itself as appreciation or even gratitude, giving rise to a 'halo effect' (Harrison, 1992: 18). Consideration of the role of the individual is particularly relevant when considering medical power. This is because of the relatively strong cohesiveness of the medical fraternity, which means that collective action may not be effective in overcoming this group due to the others' relative lack of organisation. This limitation applies not only to lay groups, but also to other health care personnel, who demonstrate, probably decreasingly, deference. Thus, medical power is exerted with the minimum of explicit conflict (Harrison, 1992: 19). This is due to any divergence being submerged, in order to avoid loss of face among the non-medical combatants should the likely defeat ensue.

The mantra which is to be expected in response to any criticism of medical high-handedness will be 'clinical freedom'. This knee-jerk reaction has the effect of warning off any who threaten to stray on to medical territory. Thus managers and midwives will, in the supposed interest of the medical relationship with patients, be cautioned about the extent of their own responsibilities (Harrison, 1992: 101). Medical power, in this way, carries with it an aura of incontestability.

A problem with medical power, which is making its survival less and less tenable, is its limitation or tunnelling of vision. Medical vision may not extend as far as the ineffectiveness of some medical practices (Illich, 1997). In addition, the move towards evidence-based practice has thrown up the unjustifiable nature of some practices (see 'Research' above) and the iatrogenic nature of others. Even worse, a series of medical scandals have shown that the medical fraternity is not actually in a position to honour its side of the bargain to keep its own house in order (Smith, 2000).

Obstetrical power

Medical power in the context of childbearing is as deeply entrenched as in any other aspect of human life, and possibly more so. This power has successfully persuaded a wide range of people of the veracity of certain highly questionable 'truths'. Examples are Cahill's (2001) report of the widespread perception of a hospital birth being the 'safe' option. Similarly, it has been argued that this perception of safety applies equally to being a benefit of having a 'doctor in control' (Bates, 1997: 134; Corea, 1977).

A further power of obstetrics lies in its pervasiveness; this is demonstrated by having infiltrated every aspect of childbearing. This pervasive power has been achieved by persuading all those involved to accept such infiltration as the norm, rather than as an aberration. Thus midwives allow themselves to be persuaded that, for example, frequent vaginal examinations in labour achieve beneficial outcomes. Such practices, due to the force of medical power, are likely to be implemented regardless of the presence or absence of the obstetrician.

A crucial aspect of obstetrical power is the phenomenon termed 'the medical gaze' (Foucault, 1963: 89). This is infinitely more than observation, compassion or the ability to provide care. The medical gaze includes 'the power of decision and intervention'. In this way the woman's co-operation is assured and the scientific credentials of the obstetric profession are established. This has been achieved by a reductionist approach to labour, involving the requirement of progress and its measurement by predefined standards. Inevitably automatic intervention ensues if and when these standards are not achieved.

The ultimate manifestation of medical power is the perception of institutionalised violence with which some women have associated medicalised childbirth. Women's interpretation of birth in this way may relate to previous experience of sexual assaults (J.V. Kitzinger, 1992). Such prior experience, however, is by no means a prerequisite for a woman to feel that her care in labour is little more than brutality (S. Kitzinger, 1992).

Medical model in maternity

The awesome power of the obstetrician in determining the care of healthy women experiencing uncomplicated childbirth is inextricably bound up with the successful and all-pervading application of the medical model. This model of childbearing prominently features the pathologisation of maternity (Scully, 1994: xviii). As Cahill (2001: 335) explains, it is due in no small part to medical organisation; that is, the provision of maternity care by specialists in women's health *problems* – the gynaecologists.

The medicalisation of the culture of childbearing is virtually indistinguishable from the medical model (Barclay *et al.*, 1989). This culture change has involved the introduction of pseudo-scientific rituals and masculine domination over women's experiences. Barclay draws on the highly appropriate example of the woman's bodily position to show this domination. Apart from the obvious inferiority of any woman in a supine position, the fact that this position is determined *for* her for the attendant's convenience and not *by* her for her own needs is crucial. Barclay goes on to draw attention to the different value system inherent in the medical model, which may be termed reductionist. The example which she uses to illustrate these differences is the medical expectation of the woman being satisfied with her birth experience if she survives and has a live, healthy baby (1989: 125).

The different value systems operating may be represented by the social model and the medical model (Wagner, 1994: 6). The dichotomy between art and science serves to demonstrate the difference, and this is exemplified by the confidence of the protagonists being directed in fundamentally different directions. The social model trusts the healthy functioning of the human body and this is manifested in the assumption of the body's competence and trustworthiness 'until proven otherwise' (1994: 37). On the other hand, the medical model adopts a more pessimistic stance. This model is based on twin assumptions; first, that the process of birth is inherently dangerous, and is only to be proven safe after its successful completion. The second, corresponding or reciprocal assumption is that technology is safe until it is shown to be dangerous. This technological aspect of the medical model has resulted in the phenomenally speedy, even over-hasty, transition from the innovation and introduction of new technologies to their routinisation (see p. 37). Wagner suggests that this process is aggravated by a 'technological imperative', comprising a perception of pressure to fully use any new equipment (1994: 7).

Of particular help in understanding the role of the medical model in maternity is the research of Scully, who studied medical attitudes among neophyte obstetricians (1994). She regards her research as having a wider application, beyond childbearing, to the extent that it serves to exemplify the development of social control throughout human society. The characteristics which Scully found to be essential to the application of the medical model are threefold.

The first is the 'distancing' which is a prerequisite for the obstetrician to be able to function effectively (1994: 102, 139). This attribute features as fundamental to the 'surgical mentality' which seeks to ignore the humanity of clients and patients.

The second characteristic identified by Scully is the focus on abnormality. For her informants healthy childbearing was of no interest whatsoever and held no attraction. Their role was to search for abnormal phenomena which would provide an opportunity for them to practise their obstetric skills (1994: 165). This pursuit and identification of problems was referred to as 'locating pathology' (1994: 220), or combining it with 'distancing', 'finding material' (1994: 219).

The third main characteristic is the display of confidence. Scully generously discusses this in terms of the medical practitioner recognising the limitations of both his own knowledge and medical knowledge. She discusses how this characteristic is of benefit to both the obstetrician and those around him. She indicates that self-confidence is necessary for his effective functioning. Scully does not, however, show the point at which the obstetrician crosses the possibly imperceptible line from being confident to becoming arrogant.

A qualitative research project on the differences between community midwives and medical staff (Pitt, 1997) further illuminates the relationship between the midwife and her medical colleagues. Broadly speaking, Pitt identified significant differences between the two groups in the contextualisation of the birth experience. Although the members of both disciplines were or had been community practitioners, the 'community' had fundamentally different meanings for the midwives and the medical practitioners. The midwives perceived themselves as part of the community and offering a service to other community members. This was exemplified by the phrase 'dinner did not matter' (1997: 222), meaning that personal matters, such as meals, came second. The medical practitioners, on the other hand, talked of 'family doctoring', meaning that childbirth offered early contact with the new family, which was effectively a 'loss leader'.

Another significant example of the differing orientation between the two groups was their attitudes to the birth of a baby with a deformity. The midwife's social focus led her, for the sake of the family, to fear deformity. The medical practitioner, on the other hand, adopted an illness focus and would be responsible for putting that baby into 'a glass jar in a pathology museum' (1997: 223). Thus the medical practitioners and the midwives were divided by their perception of the woman as a clinical object or as a social being, respectively (1997: 225).

As mentioned above (see p. 58), the medical focus is on pathology and intervening to reduce the danger which it brings. One of Pitt's respondents articulated this point in terms of intervention being the medical *raison d'être* (1997: 224). In contrast the midwife would, in the event of a problem, share the family's anxiety. This enthusiasm for intervention materialised again in the different attitudes to the duration of labour. Whereas the midwife was prepared to rely on 'nature's time', the medical practitioner resorted to 'clock time' (Pitt, 1997: 224). A further difference identified by Pitt is the way in which each group described its practice. She found that the medical practitioners used words such as 'conscious', 'anaesthetised' and 'lithotomy' (1997: 226). The midwives' knowledge, however, was more embodied, requiring her strenuous and graphic body language to clarify aspects of her practice.

A significant component of the medical model is medical language. The medical use of language has been recognised as a power ploy by many midwifery writers (Jackson and Mander, 1995; Kirkham, 1986; Shapiro *et al.*, 1983; Stephens, 1998). Both the words that are used and the setting in which they are structured serve to maintain the domination of the medical practitioner over the childbearing woman and those near her.

Conclusion

It is clear that the medical model has been applied to childbirth utterly ruthlessly and successfully. The introduction of this model has clearly had serious implications for the childbearing woman as well as for the midwife. The relative absence of the midwife in this analysis suggests that she has been comparatively passive, even acquiescent, in this process. It may be argued, therefore, that the woman has been seriously betrayed by the midwife. As both of these groups have suffered and are still suffering, it is necessary for the midwife to regain the woman's confidence so that, together, they are able to assert themselves.

Chapter 3

Fathers and fatherhood

Introduction

> Fathers and fatherhood have had a bad press in Britain over the last few years.
>
> (Burghes *et al.*, 1997: 7)

This observation may be true so far as it goes. It should, however, be added that the breadth of that bad press is narrow to the point of tunnel vision. The recent upsurge in interest in the father has focused almost exclusively on fathers with problems. The result is that this media attention has given rise to a perception of a 'crisis of fatherhood' (Gillis, 2000: 225). Thus, the fathers who are departed, deviant, deadbeat or deprived of contact have been investigated *ad infinitum* (French, 1995: 1; Marsiglio, 1995: 4). But the father who does not demonstrate such unfortunate characteristics has attracted far less research interest or media attention. In the same way, considerable attention has been focused on the father and his role at the labour and birth (see Chapter 4). It needs to be noted, though, that other aspects of the child-bearing cycle have attracted little or no interest.

In this chapter, therefore, I aim to address the research and other literature on the non-pathological aspects of fatherhood which are unconnected to the birth. The aim is to provide a general overview of fathering. This overview will serve as a foundation for the subsequent chapters on the more precise points in the man's career in relation to childbearing. In the course of this overview, it is possible that the existence and nature of the 'crisis of fatherhood' may be illuminated.

While it may be too obvious to state, it is necessary to recognise the symmetrical and possibly reciprocal relationship between motherhood and fatherhood. In this chapter, though, the assumption is being made that the reader is at least aware of the debates around motherhood. This assumption is considered to be a safe one in view of the greater media 'exposure' which has traditionally been given to motherhood (Lupton and Barclay, 1997: 1).

Recent history

The historical study of families in general and fatherhood in particular is 'bedevilled' by the limited number of sources available (McKee and O'Brien, 1982). Such study relies on primary sources such as diaries, letters, legal documents and portraits. It is difficult, though, to judge whether what we learn of the affluent families who produced these artefacts also applies to their less advantaged neighbours. Superimposed on this caution, the context of the family's life clouds the picture further. The locality, the occupation and the religion are examples of such influential contextual factors. In pre-modern times the definition of 'the family' was fiendishly complex, even when compared with its relatively fluid twenty-first-century equivalent (See below). This complexity is reflected in the historical preference for the term 'household' (Gillis, 2000). The family group has often included a wide range of resident and non-resident members who have been linked in various ways, but not necessarily either by blood or by marriage. In this strictly hierarchical arrangement the father's authority over the household may have waxed and waned, but he continued to remain powerful to the extent of being accountable only to God (McKee and O'Brien, 1982: 15). This powerful position was easily maintained in pre-industrial societies due to the location of work being either in the home or else near to it. This location facilitated men's close supervision of child-rearing activities, such as wet-nursing, infant feeding and instruction in moral and religious orientation. Thus men assumed an important educational function in the home. This is a role which was denied to women due to their supposedly more emotional demeanour (Lupton and Barclay, 1997: 37).

In the earlier part of the nineteenth century, the decades leading up to the Victorian era brought a series of changes in roles. First, parental power began to be replaced by the concept of parental duty. At the same time the hierarchical social and family relations moved in the direction of becoming more reciprocal. Second, with the industrial revolution a division of labour developed between women and men. Women's sphere became the home and men's became the paid workplace. This division, of course, was less than totally accurate as working-class women rarely worked only in the home. That was a luxury enjoyed by their upper/middle-class sisters. Although working-class men were required to labour for long hours to earn a living, their middle-class brothers were similarly absent from home in the interests of their careers. The Victorian father's stereotypical remoteness due to such absences was combined with sovereignty and moderated by benevolence (McKee and O'Brien, 1982: 18). This distance, however, has been justified by the immense pressures bearing down on the middle-class Victorian father (Tosh, 1999). While burdened with being the traditional breadwinner and protector of weak dependants, his authority was simultaneously beginning to be undermined by changing ideas about, for example, the role of women.

The strain of coping with such a dynamic situation manifested itself in his becoming distant both emotionally and physically.

The third major role change in the nineteenth century was at a fundamentally different level. These changes, according to Gillis, manifested themselves most obviously in the revolutions in France and America. These countries over-turned the patriarchal regime 'literally and symbolically' (2000: 229). Due to denying patriarchy and any other hierarchical relationships, 'citizenship' became all-important. As well as the national eradication of monarchies, personal patriarchal relationships were called into question. Gillis goes on to suggest, however, that the patriarchal family relationships were not obliter-ated, but were simply transferred into the public sphere; that is, to the means of production or business.

The variations mentioned above also characterised Edwardian fathers. The two groups to whom this breakdown in relationships applied most strongly were at the extremes; that is, the poorest and the richest members of society (McKee and O'Brien, 1982: 19). The children of such fathers had least contact with their parents because the poor survived on the streets and the rich were attended by servants. In the early twentieth century such observations gave rise to concerns about the lack of a paternal influence on both girl and boy children. These concerns became focused on the question of whether the elimination of patriarchy had overstepped the mark. The legislative process was used in Europe and in North America to correct the excesses of the nineteenth century. Because the father's presence was considered necessary to balance the mother's crucially different approach (Lupton and Barclay, 1997: 41), legislation punished what was then perceived as deviance. Thus homosexuality, non-support of families and desertion were criminalised. These legislative measures had the effect of shoring up the bourgeois norm of the father as breadwinner and endorsing the link between masculinity and fatherhood (Gillis, 2000: 230).

Thus the father's limited contact with his offspring in recent history has been appropriately summarised as being both socially and occupationally determined:

> The performance of fatherhood roles cannot be divorced from socially imposed divisions of labour which have excluded the male from the home as effectively as they have tied women to it.
>
> (Lummis, 1982: 56)

This interpretation is supported by Smith's more recent study of the father role (1995). She found that increasing numbers of UK women reported the greater likelihood of paternal involvement in certain infant care tasks between the 1950s and the 1990s. This 'task-oriented' approach, however, fails to show the extent to which the parents shared more general responsibility for child care and whether this sharing has changed.

Definitions

Differing forms of 'fatherhoods' have arisen as a result of a range of historical, societal and technological developments (Burghes *et al.*, 1997: 13; Townsend, 1999). These authors differentiate the biological father from the man who is the social or nurturing father. Whereas the former provides half of the child's genetic blueprint, the latter is usually the resident or surrogate care provider. Townsend suggests that fatherhoods, like masculinities (see p. 66 below), are subject to a multiplicity of influences, but that any variations are far less likely to be recognised as anything other than a dereliction of duty. The definitions of fatherhood assume even greater relevance, and complexity, in the context of assisted reproductive techniques. It is possible, though, that the definition of fatherhood may differ according to the discipline which is using it, depending on whether it is law, psychology, sociology, medicine, social work or social policy.

Fatherhood has also frequently been 'defined', though not necessarily in verbal form, by the use of imagery. Most memorable are the seriously macho photographic images which have recently begun to appear on calendars. Alternatively, similar macho images may be used to advertise, for example, cars or breast-feeding through postcard images. To these pictorial images may be added the fathers to whom we are frequently introduced in soap operas. One's thoughts turn to the crowd of wimpish men who inhabit Ambridge, home to *The Archers*. These visual and aural images might be easily dismissed, were it not for the close and intense attention which they are given in the relatively serious literature on fatherhood (Burgess, 1997; LaRossa, 1997; Lloyd, 1995; Lupton and Barclay, 1997).

Marsiglio suggests that these images matter so much because of the large number of young men who grow up in households in which there is no single long-term resident male (1995: 14). This means that a genuine role model is lacking for such young men and that the media version must serve as a substitute. That men really learn how to be fathers from soap operas sounds, to say the least, unlikely. This interpretation is advanced, though, by Daly (1995: 21), who cites the psychoanalytic work of Chodorow (1978). He regards the mother as the crucial person and role model in the life of the child of either gender. Even when he is resident, the father is likely to be un-available to the young man for most of his growing years due to the demands of employment. The mother, on the other hand, would be infinitely available and influential. Thus, Chodorow argues, men's parenting abilities are not fostered and may actually be diminished.

The media images of fatherhood are, for these reasons, regarded as significant. Such stereotypical images, though, may be of further, more serious significance. These other images relate to the way that the father is or is not depicted in the research literature. A good example is found in the work of Daly (1995: 26). Like many others, he found, in the course of a qualitative research project, that he encountered the widely recognised problem of recruiting male respondents. Because of men's reluctance to participate in research projects, there is a tendency for the researcher to rely on the mother's views and her interpretation of her partner's behaviour (e.g. Smith, 1995). In this way it would appear that the stereotypical images of the father have been further perpetuated (Marsiglio, 1995: 5).

Developments

There is a range of social and technological changes which may be included among the reasons for the father's 'bad press' mentioned by Burghes and colleagues (1997, above). Before exploring the nature of fatherhood, it may be helpful to examine some of the societal developments which have recently been influential in determining its nature.

Demographic and social changes

Demographic and social changes affecting fatherhood may be attributable to a variety of factors. These include the breakdown of relationships between parents and the formation of new relationships. The children of both the old and the new relationship may share accommodation, carers and providers, although their origins may differ markedly. These developments within the family have been associated with relatively recent legislative changes (Tosh, 2000: 26).

These complex family relationships, however, may not necessarily be such a modern development. When death in childbirth and other forms of early adult death were more common, complex families developed, but for different reasons. Thus declining mortality rates may have been one of the reasons for step-relationships and half-siblingships having been less prominent in the heyday of the nuclear family immediately after the Second World War. This situation, however, may have been merely a temporary aberration. The recent increasing complexity or 'blending' of families (Townsend, 1999; Walker et al., 2002) may constitute a return to the previous steady state, albeit for different reasons. These demographic changes may have been exacerbated by changes in the pattern of employment, such as the reduction in the working week which, theoretically, permits the man to spend more time with his family.

The changing role of women

The other major development which has contributed to the current interest in fathers and fatherhood is the changing role of women. The increasing labour force participation among the mothers of small children inevitably carries wide-ranging implications for the other parent. These implications may have been aggravated by the decline in certain 'heavy' industries in which only men have traditionally been employed. This decline has been negatively correlated with the growth of the service-based economy, resulting in an increasingly important role for women as breadwinners. The domestic division of labour has, in this way, been fertile ground for immense role change. The resulting need for change in child care arrangements has similarly been ripe for role reversal. Whether this potential for change has been fulfilled is a quite different matter and one which is given some attention in Chapter 5.

Masculinities

Whereas 'manhood' may have been defined relatively easily in the past, since the advent of the study of masculinities in the closing years of the twentieth century (Marsiglio, 1995: 1) such definitions have been cast into the realms of history. Because of the inevitable impact of masculinities on fatherhood, it is necessary to consider what this development comprises.

In his relatively early writing on the background to recent changes in masculinities, Seidler (1997: 1) outlines what he perceives to be the threats to the traditional masculine role. First are the threats exerted by other men, such as those who are gay. These threats give rise to hidden and unspoken anxieties among their heterosexual peers. Second are the threats exerted by feminists, which are of a similarly veiled nature; Seidler maintains that such threats are exemplified by women who seek to free themselves from the stereotypically subordinate female role, such as those women without a long-term male partner who choose to have children (1997: 10). Seidler emphasises the traditional centrality of fatherhood in establishing a man's masculine credentials. Regretting the all-too-frequent absence of the father, Seidler wonders how such sons are able to learn fathering skills. He concludes, as has been mentioned above, that figures in soap operas may be used as role models from whom to learn this function. Seidler is disdainful of the phenomenon who has become known as the 'new man', suggesting that he is little more than the answer to a marketing executives' headache.

A more enlightened view of the development of masculinities is advanced in the work of MacInnes (1998). In his critique of this area of study, MacInnes regards masculinity as synonymous with patriarchy, resulting in a perpetual crisis situation. Courtenay (2000: 1387) builds on the ideas propounded by MacInnes, by recognising the problems associated with the widely accepted stereotypes of what may be portrayed as the masculine role. Courtenay suggests that the view of men as dominant in certain societies may have been created, like a self-fulfilling prophecy, by dominant men. He disputes the traditional view of gender as a fixed or static and mutually exclusive phenomenon, arguing that there are a variety of forms of both femininity and masculinity. Courtenay suggests that there are a number of factors which influence an individual's gender role, an important example being the cultural environment, which may be combined with the location in time and place. The inevitable unpredictability of such an environment means that gender needs to be viewed as a more fluid or dynamic phenomenon than has traditionally been the case. The ways in which masculinity are demonstrated is correspondingly fluid and dynamic. It is the culture, place and time which specify the implements to be used by the masculine man, and these may be clubs, fists, guns or cars (Courtenay, 2000: 1390).

Another crucial factor which influences the manifestation of gender is the balance of power. It is recognised that the micro-level interactions between less powerful women and low-status men with the majority of men, serve to continue the macro-level subordination of the former groups. Rather than the widely assumed male on female domination, Courtenay maintains that it is the imbalance between the more and the less powerful groups which constitutes patriarchy (2000: 1388).

The conflicts arising out of the diametrically opposed views of masculinity represented by Seidler and by Courtney are addressed by Gough in his analysis of how men attempt to cope with the challenges to their traditional hegemonic role (2001). His interview-based study shows the extent to which men are vulnerable to confrontations with feminists and with unreconstructed men. In such disconcerting encounters the men whom he interviewed reported using avoidance tactics, rather than allowing open conflict to materialise.

The implications of the increasing interest in masculinities for fatherhood are manifold. One important development, though, is the change in the former emphasis on men's *duties*, which has been mentioned above. Bertola and Drakich, in introducing their work on the fathers' rights movement, indicate a move in the direction of such rights, which is comparable with men's rights and gay rights (1995: 230).

Fatherhood

As mentioned above (see Chapter 1, p. 16), fatherhood is usually better conceptualised as a social and cultural construct rather than as a biological fact of life. This observation appears to have been ignored by the multitude of legislators in Western societies who make strenuous efforts to persuade biological fathers of their social and cultural obligations (Moss, 1995: xvi). In spite of these efforts, views of the father role and fatherhood tend to be categorised along traditional and modern or 'new' lines.

Traditional fatherhood

Historians have shown that the traditions of fatherhood are long, complex and frequently mythological (Gillis, 1997). Irrespective of the origins of the perception, though, the father has traditionally been perceived as the more distant parent. These roles are summarised in terms of him being:

- An authority figure
- A disciplinarian
- A bridge between the family and the outside world
- The family breadwinner.

(Moss, 1995: xi)

These roles clearly endorse the view of the father as having his main functions outwith the domestic setting. This contrasts with the mother, whose responsibility and sphere of influence is widely perceived as lying within the home. This view of the father as the relatively remote parent is endorsed in the literature review undertaken prior to a qualitative research project on fathers' role models (Daly, 1995). This researcher recognises that the mother is traditionally regarded as the parent who is closer to the child or children by summarising the father's roles as:

- A provider
- A parent
- A source of support for the mother.

(Daly, 1995: 24)

This view of the father as being marginal to the family axis is a recurring theme, in spite of its supposedly weak origins. On the basis of his anthropological research in Botswana, Africa, and California, USA, Townsend identifies the crucial role of the mother; he describes how the father's relationships with his children are 'mediated' by the children's mother (1999: 92). He goes on to describe how the father is effectively disempowered, by means of the mother being the 'primary parent' or 'default parent' (1999: 92). Townsend continues by recounting how the woman effectively choreographs the relationships within the family, including interactions between the father and his children. This researcher's perception of family life verges on the Machiavellian when he suggests that these strategies are employed by the woman in order to maintain her own salience and that she is actually supported by the man in achieving this.

That ideas about the father role are changing or being changed is evidenced by the differing emphases in defining his role. Marsiglio introduces the concept of commitment, causing a crucial final change in direction, which serves to demonstrate movement in the direction of the 'new father':

- The breadwinner
- The moral overseer
- The sex role model
- The nurturer of the family.

(Marsiglio, 1995: 2)

These changes in perceptions of the traditional father role are found in very different sources. They show that the presence or absence and effectiveness or otherwise of the father has implications not only for sons. Writing from a feminist point of view, Barclay and Lupton suggest that even in relatively traditional relationships the father's presence is needed to 'validate' the femininity and enhance the self-esteem of girl children (1999: 1014). These researchers argue the crucial contribution of an 'external influence' on fatherhood, as opposed to the usual assumption of its being a socio-cultural construction.

'New fatherhood'

The existence of the new father will be addressed in more detail in Chapter 5, but the concept needs to be mentioned here, if only for the sake of completeness. The recognition of developments in at least the rhetoric of traditional fatherhood has been demonstrated already. The gradual move away from the father as moral teacher, through breadwinner and sex role model in the direction of the new nurturant father has been long and widely discussed (Lamb, 1986).

In spite of its long history, though, many fundamental questions still need to be asked about fatherhood. Not least is whether it is actually to become the 'loving, engaged, participative and available' phenomenon which some anticipate (Moss, 1995: xvi).

Such questions are implicit in the writing of Lupton and Barclay (1997), who describe how the 'new father' is lampooned in the media. His trademark 'baby-food stained trousers and a child hanging from each leg' are sources of derisive mirth (1997: 80). He is defined in terms of the man who is prepared to take time out from the demands of paid employment. This time is spent being nurturing and emotionally demonstrative with his children and undertaking his share of household chores. As with so many aspects of fatherhood, the media (see above) join battle. Lupton and Barclay maintain that the new father invariably suffers a worse press than his more traditional brothers.

The gap between the rhetoric and the reality of new fatherhood invariably features in this bad press (Hondagneu-Sotelo and Messner, 1994: 205). While these authors advance an economic argument to explain the existence of the gap, Segal's explanation focuses on power relations. She argues that fear of the loss of patriarchal hegemony underpins men's reluctance to increase their input into parenting (1990). Although attitudinal changes towards child care and housework appear to have begun, they have not been sufficient, or sufficiently translated into action, to manifest themselves in the reality of domestic activities.

Becoming a father

As with so many aspects of fatherhood, the crucial role of the media re-emerges with examination of the development of the father role. Whereas fatherhood is studied all too often in the context of inadequate fathering, the research by Daly (1995) focused on men becoming fathers in intact families. Using a grounded theory design he showed the effects of the absence of role models for fathering. Daly established that suitable role models were invariably lacking but that, in their absence, the men in his sample were keen to talk about their own fathers. The respondents were keen to emphasise that their fathers were not role models, but rather a point of reference or a 'jumping off point' (1995: 28). While each of the fathers denied having a role model, they did admit to having learned some activities from their own fathers. They adopted quite a narrow view of what was little more than imitation of their own fathers' behaviours. The respondent fathers did actually claim to have learned, from not having had a role model, that having one would be advantageous. For this reason the fathers in the sample expressed their enthusiasm to act as role models for their own children.

As well as the father's personal family history, his enthusiasm to adopt traditional or other fathering activities is likely to be affected by his current status. This would include, for example, his level of career establishment and the aspirations of his peer group and sexual partners (Marsiglio, 1995: 17–18). In addition, 'intrapsychic scripting' is likely to be a determining factor (Marsiglio, 1995: 78–9). This strategy involves the private construction of images of themselves. Because these images reflect their concerns about others' evaluations of them as fathers, they influence their fathering behaviour.

The father-to-be

It is clear from the discussion so far in this chapter that the concept of fatherhood is about far more than the merely biological facts of reproduction. In spite of this, while the woman is pregnant, the role of the father has been shown to matter to all concerned, including carers and researchers. Because his role at this time has recently attracted so much research as well as more general attention, it is necessary to examine now why the father is considered to be so important during pregnancy.

The father and pregnancy

It is a commonplace observation that the man's reaction to the pregnancy is different from that of the woman. Niven (1992: 14) attributes these differences to the physical experiences of the couple, such as the woman being nauseated, feeling fetal movement or needing to buy a new size of bra. The man's emotional reaction to the pregnancy, though, will vary according to a wide range of factors; these may include his cultural expectations, his experience of being loved, the nature of the couple's relationship or his confidence in his masculinity (Burdette Saunders, 1999: 211). May (1982) found that the father's reaction to his partner's pregnancy tends to follow three distinct phases. The first, the 'announcement' phase, lasts for a variable period of time from hours to weeks. During this time the father comes to accept the biological fact of the pregnancy. Depending on the circumstances, this phase may be accomplished easily or it may hold a range of challenges. The second or 'moratorium' phase is when the father begins to adjust to the reality of the pregnancy. This may extend to contemplating the spiritual meaning of the pregnancy or considering it in cosmic terms. May termed the final phase 'focusing', which comprises a wide range of largely physical preparatory activities, usually with the mother. It is at this time that the man is likely to begin to regard himself as a father. Although May's typology appears to be quite anodyne, the challenges which characterise this adaptation sometimes have a more disconcerting side. This is because they have been held responsible for the development of the couvade syndrome (see Chapter 1) as well as being blamed for the increased incidence of domestic violence during pregnancy (see Chapter 6).

The changes in the parents' relationship in association with the pregnancy may constitute one example of these challenges to the father. The increasing dependency on others, which the woman characteristically shows during pregnancy, may serve to threaten the equilibrium which a man enjoys in a relationship (Scott-Heyes, 1983). In order to study the changing relationships during and after pregnancy a questionnaire study involving seventy couples was undertaken by Scott-Heyes (1983). This study sought to ascertain the nature of the changes and the pregnancies that are 'at risk'. Scott-Heyes showed the reduction in affection in the latter part of the first pregnancy, although the level did not change with subsequent pregnancies. This study supported earlier work indicating the woman's greater dependency in pregnancy. The men's responses, though, were a cause for some concern. This is because, while a majority of the men did become more 'nurturant' (1983: 25), half of the women still considered that their needs were not being satisfied. This dissatisfaction was found to persist even after the birth. Scott-Heyes generalises her findings by suggesting that this mismatch between the woman's needs and the man's ability to both recognise and meet them may not be unique to childbearing relationships.

The stressful nature of becoming a father emerged from a quantitative study by Sullivan-Lyons (1998: 227). This researcher applied a battery of postal questionnaires to the thirty couples who were approached and agreed to participate, although the actual completion rate was nearer 70 per cent. As has been found elsewhere (see Thomas and Upton, 2000, Chapter 1, this volume), Sullivan-Lyons identified the limited extent to which the man's health symptoms, which she considered to be a psychosomatic couvade, were both recognised and dealt with. She went on to show that the instruments which are widely used to assess emotional well-being in pregnancy may not be appropriate to research involving men, on the grounds that men are less likely to report any negative feelings than are their women partners.

The difficulties which men are widely thought to experience during their partner's pregnancy have been approached from a more anthropological viewpoint by the feminist writers and researchers Lupton and Barclay (1997: 32–3). While preparing for their major qualitative study of fatherhood in Australia, these researchers studied the implications of embodiment during pregnancy. They found that women's 'leaky' bodies become even less well defined in association with childbearing. This lack of definition is attributed to the woman's sharing of her body with, first, her partner at the time of the conception, second, with her fetus during pregnancy, and third, with her baby while breast-feeding. Lupton and Barclay show the basic or primitive reactions which such sharing of the body is likely to arouse both in the woman and in her partner. These reactions are due to the loss of bodily autonomy which has been taken for granted in Western societies for at least three centuries. While women are relatively comfortable with the 'leakiness' of their bodies, each one having experienced it at least since her menarche, her male partner is likely to be less comfortable with it. These authors go on to suggest that women's expectations of bodily autonomy may be lower than men's. In support of this, examples are provided of men's need to exert control over women's childbearing bodies. These examples include enforced sterilisation, intrauterine surgery and criminalising pregnant drug users; to which should be added court-ordered caesarean (see Weaver, 2002, Chapter 2, this volume). This, often judicial, control may be translated into individuals' behaviour by men who avoid 'women's work' with converting fluids into solids, such as washing, butter-making and cooking. More extreme examples would include men's abhorrence of leakiness, such as tears, or other fluidity in their own bodies. Thus the man's bodily hardness and dryness verges on becoming a *raison d'être*. These feminist writers' profound insights into the male anxieties relating to childbearing demonstrate the fundamental difficulties which men are likely to face in association with a partner's pregnancy.

In a large and significant study, Draper (2002) succeeded in identifying some of these fundamental difficulties. The aim of Draper's project was to study men's views of their transition to fatherhood. Her ethnographic study involved the easy recruitment of eighteen men from National Childbirth Trust classes. She then undertook focus groups and individual face-to-face interviews. Like Lupton and Barclay (1997), Draper found that embodiment featured prominently in this man's experience. In her sample, though Draper found that it was 'his inability to directly experience the embodied nature of the pregnancy' (2002: 265) that caused the man to perceive that he was too detached from the pregnancy. This was one of the reasons why the man found difficulty achieving the involvement which he craved.

The other reason for the men in Draper's sample experiencing difficulty was even less tangible. This reason related to the different sources of knowledge accessed and used by women and men. Obviously, the men's partners were able to draw on their embodied knowledge of the pregnancy through their intimate relationship with the fetus. Such knowledge is generally denied to men, although one of them reported his fervent appreciation of being privileged to experience the movement of the fetus:

M: I found the feeling of the baby moving to be much more exciting than the scan.
RESEARCHER: Why do you think that was?
M: I don't know . . . I suppose it's because the scan was a machine.
(Draper, 2002: 568)

This exchange demonstrates a learning curve for the man which is steep to the extent of being vertical. The reason is the tendency of men to stereotypically favour knowledge which is based on science and measurement. Women, on the other hand, are content to rely on knowledge which originates in human beings and their feelings. In this context these would include, for example, fetal movements as well as 'old wives' tales'. Draper describes graphically how the men in her sample were forced to 'wrestle' (2002: 567) with these two sources of knowledge. Draper contends that maternity care, due to medicalisation, tends to rely more heavily on the masculine, objective forms of knowledge. The men were more comfortable with these objective aspects of the pregnancy, such as confirmation by pregnancy testing. On the basis of her findings, Draper recognises the importance to the father of 'body-mediated-moments', such as confirmation, the scan and the labour.

The father and childbirth education

The notion that childbirth education might be of help to men in facing the challenges of their partners' pregnancy is relatively novel. The traditional assumption has been made that men need no preparation for such a limited role. This is because fathers have been permitted to enter the labour ward only on condition that they are of help to their partner and do not upset the labour area's smooth functioning. That the father might have his own personal needs and paternal reasons for being involved has rarely been taken into account. Clearly, this situation is far from ideal if the breadth of fatherhood and the challenges of becoming a father, as discussed above, are taken into account. The research into the father's childbirth education experience has only approached a limited number of relatively specific aspects of childbearing. Most of these have sought only to address the role of the father when the woman is in labour (Bennett *et al.*, 1985; Bertsch *et al.*, 1990; Chapman, 1992; Greenhalgh *et al.*, 2000).

An attempt to overcome this deficiency in the literature was made by Nolan (1994). By undertaking a survey of thirty fathers attending classes with six NCT (National Childbirth Trust) teachers, Nolan aimed to discover what men seek in the classes and the nature of their worries about pregnancy and labour. A six-point questionnaire was given to all of the fathers prior to the first class and collected before the class started, resulting in a 100 per cent response rate. The responses related to the men's needs for factual information about the labour and child care. A rating scale to assess the importance of the topics earned the highest score (289/300) for 'Helping my partner in labour'. The lowest score went to 'Sexuality in pregnancy and after the birth', which earned only 136/300.

On the basis of these findings, Nolan claims that she had identified 'what men want from their antenatal classes' (1998: 147). Included in what men are concerned about, she maintains, is 'Their own adjustment to fatherhood' (1994: 28). While this would be a most appropriate concern, this topic is not mentioned in the data provided in the article; further there is no mention of the man's preparation for fatherhood. Although in the rating scale 'Caring for the baby in first few weeks' earned the relatively high score of 263/300, child care does not really equate with fatherhood. Thus this survey's findings, yet again, fail to move beyond his role in supporting his partner, particularly in labour.

Nolan's work corresponds with the findings of Smith's study of 'antenatal classes and the transition to fatherhood' (1999b, 1999c). Smith interviewed eighteen male volunteers who had attended a variety of childbirth education classes. The interviews were all held when the baby was at least two weeks old and the data were analysed qualitatively. The men were drawn from a comparatively narrow socio-economic band, as demonstrated by the fact that a large majority (78 per cent, n = 14) were graduates. It may be that this sample is an accurate reflection of the people who attend for childbirth education.

The overriding impression from this research report is the disconcertingly low expectations of the fathers of the 'classes'. Although each of the fathers was 'adamant' (Smith, 1999c: 463) that he had attended of his own free will, he had no expectation that the classes would offer him anything as a father or that the father's needs would be addressed. The expectations were totally built around the father's role as supporter to his partner, with his attendance signifying supportive commitment, rather than any enthusiasm for learning about fatherhood. Smith provides a useful insight into the man's role in childbearing, which supports the findings of Draper (2002, above), when she reports her finding that each of the men felt 'safer' (Smith, 1999c: 465) with the technical information which the classes provided.

Each of the men in this study said that they were happy to be 'in the back seat' (ibid.) with regard to childbearing matters, due to the biological facts of life. This phrase, which featured prominently, indicated the father's perception of his secondary role and that learning about childbearing was essentially 'women's business' (1999c: 463). The father distinguished parenthood, which he considered to be crucially important, from fatherhood, which he could not define and was of far lower priority. Smith found that the men she interviewed fell into three groups: the 'totally committed', the 'passive accepter' or the 'reluctant attender'. The data showed that the individual men moved between the three groups, which Smith attributes to the nature of the classes which they attended.

This unfortunate impression of the father's attendance without involvement reflects the observation which Barbour made in 1990 on the basis of her research with parents over the complete childbearing cycle. Her anticipation, that fathers' consolidation of their position in the labour ward would be extended to the postnatal period, does not appear to have materialised.

The work of Nolan (1998) and Smith (1999b, 1999c) suggests that the father has little understanding of the magnitude of fatherhood and that this incomprehension is reflected in his preoccupation with the minutiae of child care and the technology of childbirth. An attempt to extend the man's vision beyond the practical details, by using childbirth education, was made in a Wisconsin-based study (Diemer, 1997). The aim was to benefit the father and, indirectly, the family by teaching the father interpersonal skills which were intended to reduce the stress of new parenthood. This quasi-experimental study involved two groups of expectant couples, making a total of 108 couples. Forty couples completed the 'traditional' series of classes and forty-three couples completed the experimental or 'father-focused' series. The class for the 'father-focused' series was often divided into men and women to permit the fathers to 'share feelings and concerns and combat their sense of isolation by facilitating peer support' (Diemer, 1997: 286). The following topics featured prominently:

- Fathers' involvement
- Communication of feelings and caring
- Changes in male roles
- Concerns about providing financial and physical support
- Giving and receiving emotional support
- Sexuality
- Pregnancy and parenting.

The post-test results did not show the significant differences which the researchers had anticipated. The data showed, though, that the man in the experimental group's likelihood of using social support had increased more than the man in the traditional group. The relationship between the partners improved similarly. The researchers recognise the difficulty of changing an established culture of parenting, and question whether such change is possible in the absence of prominent role models.

Conclusion

This all too brief consideration of fatherhood in relation to pregnancy has demonstrated the perception of the massive change which is currently pervading this topic. This perception has emerged strongly in the research and other literature from a variety of countries and disciplines.

That fatherhood is changing should come as no surprise, given the immense societal developments which inevitably impinge on the role of the father. These contextual changes include the women's movement and the long-standing changes in women's employment practices. For the man, changes in employment prospects and the nature of the work available have cast a long shadow over his roles. The advent of gay rights and the study of masculinities have had many implications which may not have been anticipated. Legislative, combined with societal, changes have affected the nature and structure of the family. In view of this wide range of awesome developments it would be surprising if fatherhood had not undergone radical modification. That fatherhood has managed to adjust to accommodate the contextual developments may be a sign of its health, rather than the reverse.

A less optimistic view of the development of fatherhood appears in the psychoanalytical writing of Gertrud Mander (2001). While observing the variable nature of fatherhood, she writes almost regretfully of the demise of the patriarchal family structure. She attributes its demise to a series of worldwide conflicts, which have removed men from the family on a shorter or a longer term basis. Thus, the woman has been required to assume the responsibilities of her partner, both within the home as well as outside it. Not surprisingly, this experience has altered the woman's self-perception and her aspirations. Mander moves on to consider, from a Freudian perspective, the nature of the man's relationships within the family. Inevitably she finds that Oedipal theories are no longer relevant, in view of the limited experience of the young person of having two cohabiting parents. Continuing to draw on Greek mythology, she suggests that Oedipal comparisons have been replaced by Olympian associations, that is, with Zeus. She applies this comparison particularly to the father's lack of commitment to the concept widely known as 'family values' (2001: 146).

This dismal impression of fatherhood has given rise in some circles to the perception of a 'crisis of fatherhood' (Gillis, 2000: 225). This North American writer attributes the origins of the decline in fatherhood to the societal changes of the 1960s. The particular aspects of the 1960s which are responsible, he maintains, are not the drug culture or the women's movement, but the economic cycle. This has meant that, due to the power of capitalism, heavy industry has been relocated in Third World countries. The result is that the 'breadwinner' role has been downgraded to employment in a service industry, or has even been assumed by the woman of the family.

It may be argued that this view is a uniquely North American perspective and that the industrial, economic and political developments have been accepted with less trauma in other countries. In spite of this, the North American artefact, which is known as the 'crisis of fatherhood', has been exported in its entirety to other countries and societies. In many of these situations the relevance of this dogma is, to say the least, questionable. Perhaps because of the importation of this dogma the father faces some degree of uncertainty about his role. This may be manifested as an acquiescence to some involvement in pregnancy care through childbirth education. The extent to which it affects his involvement in the later stages of the childbearing cycle are addressed in the following two chapters.

Chapter 4

The labour and the birth

Thus far I have examined the role of the father and male childbirth attendants in different societies, at different times and the father's role during pregnancy. This chapter aims to bring together the ideas which have already been introduced and to focus them on one particular episode in the childbearing cycle. This is the time which is widely and appropriately regarded as most momentously significant – the labour and the birth. For the woman, the significance of these events is attributable to the physical and emotional challenges which they present. To the man who is present at and involved with the labour and the birth, the challenges are likely to be equally real, but inevitably very different. The ideas from the earlier chapters are used as the foundation to focus, first, on the parents' views of the father's entry into the birthing room. This priority is appropriate because the parents are, or should be, the lead players at the birth. Second, the focus is on whether and to what extent care in labour has changed and is changing. The factors which have influenced any changes in the care provided during labour are analysed. This chapter concludes with a brief overview of the role of the male actors in the introduction of any changes which may have occurred.

The parents' views of the father's presence at the birth

As with so many interventions which are introduced into the health care system, the father's appearance and acceptance in the labour room preceded any research to evaluate the potential implications of his presence. The literature on this topic was initially solely anecdotal. Published material on the father's perception pre-dated anything purporting to present the woman's perspective. Because of this chronological arrangement, I consider here the father's views first.

The father's perception

In Chapter 1 I included a brief outline of the entrance of the father into the labour room (see pp. 33–4). This short sketch indicates some of the obstacles which the pioneering fathers found blocking their ingress. These obstacles are chronicled by Backwell in the form of a blow-by-blow account of his experience while his partner was in labour (1977). Although his perception of the atrocious behaviour of the maternity staff is abundantly clear, this account is totally devoid of any trace of this man's personal engagement with the child's birth. The only indication that this man experienced any emotional reactions to the birth of their son is his occasional reference to his incensed responses to the staff's abysmally unprofessional conduct.

Just over ten years after Backwell's ground-breaking account, the same journal published another father's narrative of the birth of Sophie, a father's first daughter (Barr, 1988). The story of Sophie's birth lacks the impotent rage of its predecessor, which seems to have been replaced with a slightly melancholy humour. Instead of the focus on the appalling behaviour of the staff, the emphasis is on the technology, such as machinery, alarms, drips and monitors. The duration of labour features, as does the perception of the associated risk. The eventual birth by caesarean operation brings with it a sense of *déjà vu*. The most glaring similarity, though, between these two men's experiences is the almost total omission of any human emotions on the part of either of these fathers. It may be that for some reason these men adopted differing strategies to achieve the same end. While Backwell joined battle with the staff, Barr was concentrating on the technology of the labour in order, presumably, to exclude the stereotypically 'unmanly' feelings and behaviour which the birth of a baby brings to those who are involved.

A more recent father's account suggests that not much has changed. McCracken's story of his son's birth, written in 1999, has more in common with Backwell's than Barr's experience. Like his predecessor by twenty-five years McCracken expresses only anger towards the medical staff who managed to transform the birth of his son into an extraction from his partner's 'belly':

> 'I still feel the inner rage build'
> 'What gets my ire the most . . . .'
> (McCracken, 1999)

Because of his continuing anger, McCracken has embarked on a crusade aimed at providing the birth experience which the couple seek, rather than the 'medical marvel' which is all too often the case.

Thus the message which arises out of this small but diverse sample of fathers' published anecdotal accounts is slightly surprising. These accounts suggest that the man's view of his experience is unconnected to either his relationship with his partner or to the child who is about to be born. These fathers demonstrate the stereotypically masculine characteristics of slightly unfocused anger and profound interest in technology. Whether the research into the father's perceptions of his experience shows differences or similarities will be addressed below.

Research into the father's perceptions

The presence of the father in the birthing room is a recent development which, I have suggested above (see pp. 33–4), reverses the long-standing, if not natural, order of things. Perhaps for this reason, as well as the messages from the plethora of anecdotal accounts mentioned above (see p. 79), the father's experience has attracted considerable attention in the research literature and other publications.

An early and important example of a qualitative study of the father's presence at the birth was undertaken in two maternity units in England by Elizabeth Perkins (1980). The 'glossy handbooks' (1980: 2), which set out the unit policy of welcoming the partner into the labour room, were contrasted with the researcher's observation of the father's limited acceptance there. Perkins identified certain well-defined roles which the father was able to perform. The first was his presence, which often served little more than to prevent the woman from having to spend long periods in labour quite alone. The second role was the father's physical contact, although this was not as straightforward as it may sound. Problems were encountered due to the arrangement of furniture in the labour room, and to the father not being given 'permission' to rearrange it. Thus even eye contact between the couple may not have been possible, even less physical contact. Perkins categorised a third role as performing 'simple nursing' tasks (1980: 21), such as giving the woman water to drink and applying wet flannels. A fourth role involved assistance with pain control; examples were back-rubbing, encouraging breathing and relaxation, and the inhalation of nitrous oxide and oxygen. On the basis of her observations, Perkins goes on to suggest how the man might be taught to perform these four tasks more effectively. The focus of this study is on the man's helpfulness towards, first, his partner and, second, the staff. Although his needs receive only scant attention, the person who appears to be most concerned about his situation is, perhaps not surprisingly, the woman in labour (1980: 24).

A similar view of the father in the labour room was reflected in the research findings recounted by Bedford and Johnson (1988). While the studies to which these writers refer, such as Cronenwett and Newmark (1974), reflected the positive nature of the father's experience, there was no detail as to why the father felt so satisfied with his presence at the birth. Bedford and Johnson summarise the then extant research findings in terms of the father's perception of his role as 'guiding and comforting' his partner and 'providing protection and familiarity in the alien hospital environment' (1988: 192). This rather limited view of the value of the father's presence resurfaces in these authors' recommendations for the improvement of the father's role. They suggest that his attendance at antenatal classes would improve matters by enabling him 'to play a major role as a coach through labour and delivery' (1988: 194).

Although Bedford and Johnson (1988) do not refer to the work of Woollett and her colleagues (1982), the similarity of the conclusions suggests that the view that the father's presence served only to benefit the woman was prevalent then. On the basis of a retrospective study and an observational study, Woollett and her colleagues suggest that the father's presence achieves three ends which they list in ascending order of priority:

- Support and assistance to the mother
- Encouraging relaxation in the mother
- Enhancement of the emotional quality of the experience for the mother.

(Woollett *et al.*, 1982: 75)

Following their observational study, which noted the new father's interactions with their newborn children, Woollett and her colleagues suggested that the significance of his presence at the birth in the formation of the father–child relationship had been overestimated (1982: 87). These researchers consider at length the difficulties which the father may face in being present at the birth. These include the attire which he is required to put on, and the extent to which this may be seen to reflect his lowly status. This authoritative work, however, makes no mention of any personal or emotional needs which the father may bring with him. Even less is there any indication of how these needs may be met by staff.

A move in the direction of at least recognising and possibly meeting the father's unique needs is found in one example of the relatively early literature on the father's experience (Brown, 1982). This study comprised interviews with fathers before and after the birth of a first child and then with 'medical and nursing staff' (1982: 105). Brown's interviewees accepted that one purpose of the father's presence was for him to 'experience the experience with his wife' (1982: 117). Although not a great step, this is a recognition that the father is at least something other than a less than satisfactory substitute for a member of staff.

The persistent focus on the father as little more than another assistant in the childbirth scenario may still be with us. This is evident in a widely welcomed qualitative study (Nichols, 1993) in which forty-four first-time fathers were questioned about the paternal behaviours which they considered to have been most useful to their partners during the birth. This North American researcher evaluated the father's activity during labour merely in terms of valuing more highly the man who was able to offer more assistance to the woman in labour.

A postal survey organised by the Royal College of Midwives sought to find an answer to the question of whether men were being 'forced into the delivery room against their wishes' (Macmillan, 1994; RCM, 1995a). The distribution of the questionnaires was slightly less than orthodox, with five questionnaires being distributed by each of the 233 RCM branches. The response rate was only 38 per cent. Ninety-eight per cent of the men who responded planned to attend the birth, but only 88 per cent denied being under pressure to be present. Thus 10 per cent of the men appear to attend the birth against their wishes, if not their better judgement. As mentioned above, the reactions of the men were largely positive. Perhaps surprisingly, though, only 68 per cent admitted to being 'pleased to be involved'. Negative feelings such as 'tired', 'scared' or 'useless' were experienced by 42 per cent, 29 per cent and 14 per cent of the men respectively. Other negative emotions, such as 'upset', 'in the way', 'not important', 'sick' or 'ignored', were articulated by smaller numbers. Unfortunately, there is no way to find out whether the 62 per cent of fathers who were given questionnaires but decided not to return them are in any way different from the fathers who did respond. It may not be surprising that the extent to which the men's needs were addressed was not able to be identified in such a survey.

The lack of research into the father's needs during the birth manifests itself in an article by Bartels (1999). She admits that 'Very little is currently known about the man's experience during shared childbirth' (1999: 681). This sorry state is endorsed by a more authoritative review of the literature (Draper, 1997). Having explored the existing literature, Draper concludes that staff influence the father's expectation of his role and, effectively, create a self-fulfilling prophecy. Although expectations are initially high, the staff effectively diminish his expectations of what the father is able and permitted to contribute during the labour and birth. The result is that his role is restricted to that of a 'labour coach' (1997: 136). Draper implies that this diminution of expectations and role is linked to the non-recognition of and non-attendance to the father's psychological and other independent needs. The evidence of the anecdotal accounts (see p. 79) endorses the existence of this downward spiral of expectations. The anecdotes indicate that the father does not perceive that his experience of the birth requires anything other than minor adjustments in staff behaviours. The absence of authoritative research in this area may, however, be being corrected. A small number of well-designed studies have recently been undertaken in Western Europe which may serve to inform the experience of the father.

The couple's expectations of each other during the birth were investigated by a qualitative study in Hampshire, England (Somers-Smith, 1999). This researcher undertook semi-structured interviews with eight couples, interviewing each member of the couple separately both before and after the birth. The woman anticipated that her partner would provide support of a practical nature, such as applying cooling cloths. His emotional support, however, was expected to be of even greater value. Prior to the birth the father found difficulty in defining the specific help which he would be able to offer and tended to fall back on describing his contribution in terms of being a 'familiar face' (1999: 104). This research identified the profound anxieties which the man experiences in this situation. His anxieties relate to matters which go as deep as the perceived threat to the survival of his partner: 'the extreme of her dying through childbirth which you hear of' (Mr C, first interview, 1999: 104). On the other hand, and at a less profound level, the man's recognition of his own considerable limitations featured prominently: 'I'll be completely shooting in the dark' (Mr H, first interview, 1999: 104).

In the interviews after the birth the men in the study were found to have come round to the women's expectations of providing more practical forms of support by the time of the labour. These men, like the Hong Kong sample reported by Ip (2000), were surprised when the woman in labour rejected this practical form of help when it was really emotional support that was being sought. The father found that he was required to provide emotional support of an intensity that he was hardly aware existed and certainly had not anticipated would be expected of him. His difficulty in being so intensively supportive was aggravated by his own anxieties and his other negative feelings, which he felt he was forced to conceal. This dual role proved challenging, especially in view of the paradox of the father being required to engage emotionally at an unexpectedly profound level while simultaneously trying to hide his anxiety, guilt and 'feelings of uselessness' (1999: 105).

On the basis of these data, it is apparent that Somers-Smith (1999) was able to identify the depth of the feelings which the father encounters during the labour and the birth of the baby. These feelings originate with general, unfocused anxiety. During the latter part of pregnancy, though, they become focused on the essentially practical aspects of helping the woman. When the woman is in labour the father's anxiety is further transformed into concern about his own emotional functioning while providing unexpectedly intense support. Thus it seems that Somers-Smith's work suggests that the father may never actually be permitted or have the opportunity to contemplate his own emotional needs around the time of becoming a father.

Whereas Somers-Smith focused mainly on the supportive nature of the father's presence, two Finnish researchers used the concept of fatherhood as their theoretical framework (Vehvilainen-Julkunen and Liukkonen, 1998). These researchers sought to question the fathers, first, about their feelings during childbirth, second, about the meaning of his presence and, third, about any changes needed in midwifery care. The questionnaire which was used comprised a Likert-type scale with a few open questions. Data were collected by handing the questionnaire to a non-random sample of fathers within two hours of the birth; it was to be returned before the woman's discharge about two to three days after the birth. Of the 132 eligible fathers who agreed to participate, 107 returned a completed questionnaire, giving the surprisingly high response rate of 81 per cent. The sample in this study included both first-time fathers (n = 47, 44 per cent) as well as fathers having a subsequent baby (n = 60, 56 per cent).

The Finnish fathers identified many pleasant as well as less pleasant aspects of being present at the birth. Their major concerns related to whether the woman was able to cope, their own feelings of helplessness, their uncertainties and their worries about the baby's welfare. The pleasant feelings included pride in their fatherhood and the baby, and gratitude to and love for their partner. Criticisms of the labour room environment and the staff also emerged.

An open item sought to identify the 'best thing' in the experience (1998: 14). A large majority of the fathers responded to this item (83 per cent), of whom most mentioned some aspect of the baby. Unlike other studies, this Finnish study was successful in being able to probe the father's feelings about any association between his presence at the birth and his fatherhood. The moment of the birth and the immediate care of the newborn baby was immensely significant to becoming a father. Each of the fathers appreciated the opportunity to be with the baby at this time and considered that it was crucial to their developing fatherhood.

Another open item asked the fathers what the hardest part of the experience had been. Again 83 per cent of the fathers responded, for whom seeing their partner in pain was considered to be the most difficult aspect (1998: 14). Highly significantly, each of these fathers felt that his difficulty in seeing her in this distressed state was aggravated by his total inability to help her by removing the pain (1998: 15). In the Likert scale some of the fathers admitted to feeling guilty about their partner's pain. It is unclear, though, whether this guilt refers primarily to the father perceiving himself as having contributed in some way to the pain or to his complete inability to remove it. Vehvilainen-Julkunen and Liukkonen suggest in the discussion that the father may perceive the pain as more painful than the woman does, implying that this may exacerbate the father's feelings of both guilt and impotence. This problem resurfaced when the questionnaire asked about any changes which might be necessary in midwifery practice. Presumably because of the difficult feelings that the fathers had encountered in response to their partner's pain, they recommended that more needed to be done to ensure adequate pain control for the woman in labour. The problem of the father's difficulty in coping with the woman's pain is an issue which will resurface later in this chapter (see pp. 93–5).

A Swedish study by Hallgren and her colleagues (1999) was undertaken as part of a larger study of the Swedish form of socialised health and maternity care. A hermeneutic phenomenological approach was used. The researchers undertook three interviews (two during the pregnancy and one after the birth) with each of eleven men whose partners were pregnant for the first time. The interviews were loosely structured, with the fathers being asked to talk about their 'expectations and experiences' of childbirth preparation and childbirth.

In spite of each of these fathers having been well prepared for the experience of childbirth, each still regarded himself as not really being ready for the event itself. The researchers found that the concept which arose out of this study was 'vital involvement', meaning that the father had a crucial role to play in the pregnancy and the childbirth and that it was an immensely active role. Although this concept reflects the father's fundamentally positive feelings about his experience of the birth, it does not give any impression of the unreadiness of the father to cope with the multiplicity of demands which the labour brings with it. Almost invariably the fathers in this research project commented that their experience of being with their partner in labour was far more demanding than they had expected.

Some of the findings resulting from these recent research projects have been raised in the context of a review article by Hall (1993). She highlights the problem, raised in many of the studies, of a man being faced with a partner who is enduring labour pain. She graphically describes how he, rather unusually, finds himself in a situation about which he is able to do absolutely nothing. She describes the effect of this impotence on the man as being 'devastating'. Hall goes on to discuss the implications which such an experience may have on the man's sexual functioning. Hall also recognises the problem of the social pressure on the man to conform with his peers who have attended the birth of their own children. She argues that the pioneering fathers may have overcome a great barrier in gaining admittance to the labour room. It is possible, Hall maintains, that the pendulum may have swung too far in the opposite direction. What this means is that the couple may be perceptive enough to realise that the father's presence at the birth will be helpful to neither of them, but that the societal expectations or pressure for him to remain with her in labour may be too overpowering for them to withstand. Hall's remarkable insight into the couple's situation seems to contribute to our understanding of the conspiracy which enforces the man's continuing presence.

The woman's perspective

It may be because women's behaviour has not changed to the same extent as men's that women's views about the father's presence in labour have attracted comparatively little research attention. The research on the mother's views which has been published, however, is generally favourable towards the father's presence and positive about his contribution.

An example of the mother's generally favourable attitude towards the father's presence is found in the study completed in England by Somers-Smith (1999). This qualitative study showed the great value which the mother attaches to the father's presence. He was found to be able to provide practical help, as well as simply being present. Somers-Smith suggests that the father may have been welcomed by virtue of the woman's perception of him taking control, although whether his presence actually allowed the mother to retain control is uncertain. The woman was also found to value the opportunity to criticise her partner in a way that she was not able to criticise the staff. As mentioned above (see pp. 80–5) the father was less than overwhelmingly positive about his experience, admitting to the stressful nature of his un-accustomed role. In relation to this stress, Somers-Smith suggests that a vicious circle may develop due to the father's mounting stress being visible to the woman. The woman's anxiety may, as a result, escalate and exacerbate her demands on her increasingly over-stressed partner (1999: 107).

Another example of the mother's satisfaction with the father's presence is found in a North American study (Entwistle and Doering, 1981). These researchers compared the experiences of women whose partner was present at the birth with those whose partner was not. Entwistle and Doering found that the presence of the partner is associated with a great enhancement of the woman's emotional experience of the birth. They go on to conclude that the presence of her partner is the cause of this enhancement and that his presence is beneficial for the woman. Researchers such as Cogan and colleagues have suggested that this finding of benefit applies more precisely to the woman's perception of labour pain (1976). Unfortunately, other researchers, such as Wallach (1982), have been unable to support these find-ings. They have even gone so far as to indicate that certain unpleasant components of labour pain may actually be aggravated if the partner is present.

Because of the uncertainty about the meaning of these conflicting findings, Niven (1985) undertook an important research project involving ninety-eight women in labour. Of these women seventy-nine were accompanied by a partner. By measuring pain levels in labour and recalled perceptions post-natally and comparing the accompanied and unaccompanied groups, Niven sought to ascertain whether the partner's presence made any difference. She found that there was no significant difference in the perception of the severity of labour pain between the accompanied women and the unaccompanied women.

Niven, however, did find that the women were generally keen to recount their satisfaction with their partner's presence and his functioning. This satisfaction applied regardless of whether he was very attentive to her and active in his ministrations or whether he was more disinterested and detached from all that was happening to her. The satisfied woman usually reported his presence as being 'comforting', that he was 'familiar' and that she was able to hold on to him. Some of the most active fathers were commended for their ability to direct or facilitate the woman's pain control or coping strategy. There was a small proportion of women who regarded him as unhelpful. Each of the women in this group maintained that she was concerned about his becoming upset by being with her while she was experiencing labour pain. On the basis of these findings, Niven concludes that the couple should be encouraged to make their own individual decisions about the father's presence and that the societal and other pressures to conform should be reduced.

The experience of the woman of having her partner present during her labour is analysed critically by Jackson (1997). Like Niven, Jackson reports the potential for the man to be traumatised by his presence at the birth, which may be a serious source of concern for the woman. Reference is also made to the possibility of the couple's sexual relationship being adversely affected by the 'battlefield' experience (Jackson, 1997: 682). Both the short-term and the long-term implications for the woman become abundantly clear. While Jackson's argument is persuasive up to this point, her reference to the rather dubious 'doula' studies, namely to recommend that the partner should be supplanted by an unqualified woman attendant, is somewhat less than convincing (G. Mander, 2001).

An anthropological view of the childbearing situation is provided by the work of Vincent-Priya (1992). She reports, as in Chapter 1 (this volume), the traditional exclusion of the father from the birth in many societies. She maintains also that the reverse traditional arrangement may apply, in which only the father and a ritual specialist may be permitted to be present. Against this background, Vincent-Priya appraises the effect of the father's presence on the woman's control over her birthing experience. She concludes that the increasing trend towards encouraging the father's presence has the effect of reducing the woman's choices (1992: 78). Vincent-Priya's conclusion may resonate with Jackson's, in that the father's presence serves to reduce the likelihood that the woman may be able to choose to have an experienced, familiar and supportive woman with her. The observation made by Vincent-Priya is reminiscent of the 'policy' of some UK maternity units, where only one person is permitted to accompany the woman in labour and it is preferred that that person is her male partner.

Thus an argument may be developing that the father's presence may not invariably be in the best interests of the woman. This argument has famously, perhaps notoriously, been taken to its logical conclusion by Odent (1999). A latter-day obstetric *enfant terrible*, he has succeeded in cornering the market in childbirth heresies. His anti-orthodoxy has endeared him to the active birth movement, with little thought for the consequences. Odent has sought to 'introduce' the gospel of non-intervention that the midwife has, when permitted, been practising for centuries. The gospel according to Michel Odent focuses on the need of the woman to withdraw into herself when in labour and 'reduce the activity of her neocortex' (1999: 23). This withdrawal is said to permit her body to give birth without the impedimenta of intellectual interference. In this way, Odent argues, the woman's hormonal activity is stimulated, the physical structures relax and cease to obtrude, and powerful uterine contractions bring about the birth of the baby.

He has termed this series of events the 'fetus ejection reflex' (Odent, 1987), indicating its similarity to a range of fundamentally profound human responses which happen quite spontaneously unless impeded by intellectual or other interference.

The interference against which Odent rails is twofold. The first is the ministrations of his obstetrical colleagues. These begin with the hospitalisation of birth, include the medicalisation of midwifery, technological interference in labour, pharmacological pain control and surgical birth, and end with evidence-based midwifery and medical practice.

The other, second *bête noire* with which Odent wrestles metaphorically is the woman's male partner – the baby's father. The father's anxiety, he contends, 'is contagious' (1999: 23), and infects the woman and impedes the complete achievement of her birthing reflex. Odent states that if the father is absent for even a short time, the impediment which he constitutes may be overcome and the birth completed physiologically. He cites 'a certain number of births' (1999: 23) in which the progress of the woman's labour has escalated as the father has departed briefly and has been completed prior to his return. Odent regards the father as fundamentally a distraction which hinders the progress of labour. Like others (see Jackson, 1997, above), Odent is concerned about the effects of the father's presence at the birth on the couple's sexual relationship. He extends this concern to attribute the rising tide of marital disharmony to the father attending the birth.

Although Odent's analysis of the problem of the father's presence has much to recommend it, the solution may be less easily identified. The solution which Odent advocates invariably comprises Michel Odent, as he features prominently in any of his material. In so doing Odent may justifiably be criticised for merely replacing one medicalised form of birth with another, even though his version of medicalisation includes fewer technological fixes. The birthing pool may replace the obstetric bed and the singing lessons may replace the syntocinon, but the coercion still serves to limit the opportunity for the woman to opt out of the style of birth for which she has originally signed up.

The impression which this brief review of the literature on the woman's perspective leaves is quite clear. The anxieties which her partner's presence cause her are overwhelmed by the woman's appreciation of his company. This conclusion is not entirely convincing, though, because the birthing woman's view has not, up until this time, been given the attention it both deserves and needs.

The staff perspective

It is clear that the view of the father about his presence at the birth has been well addressed through anecdotes and research. The mother's view of his presence has received less attention, but this deficiency is beginning to be remedied. While the initial opposition to the father's presence in terms of increasing infection, lawsuits and syncope is well documented (Cronenwett and Newmark, 1974), research into the views of maternity staff is notable by its absence or, at least, deficiency. A notable exception to this observation is found in the work of Brown (1982) which, though dated, carries important messages which may still be relevant. Angela Brown interviewed first-time fathers before and after the birth and also 'medical and nursing staff' (1982: 105). In 1980 she interviewed a sample of the labour ward staff including one nursing officer, four sisters, five staff midwives, three registrars and five consultant obstetricians.

She found, like the researchers mentioned above, that the fathers articulated their feelings of helplessness, being a hindrance, and surprise at the length and challenging nature of labour. The medical staff recognised the attempts made consciously and deliberately by the 'nursing staff' to reduce such negative reactions in the fathers. Brown reports the midwife's success in relating to the father in comparison with the efforts of the medical personnel. She seems to find this medical limitation surprising, taking account of the factors common to the fathers and the medical practitioners, such as gender and parental status. Brown found that the entire hospital staff were prepared to admit the benefits of the father's presence in facilitating a more satisfying experience of birth.

The medical staff's concerns about the father's presence focus on their uncertainty about his role in the labour room. This was articulated by all of the medical interviewees in terms of his intrusiveness in disrupting the medical status quo. While being generally perceived as 'pressure' (1982: 112), his intrusiveness was occasionally specified more precisely, such as his effect on 'the process of [medical] decision-making' (1982: 111).

Perhaps surprisingly, of particular discomfort to the medical staff was their assumption of the sexual nature of the relationship between the couple. Because of the medical staff's 'own masculinity' they were uncomfortable undertaking certain intimate tasks, such as vaginal examination, in the presence of the husband. This clearly indicates the medical perception of the sexual connotations of obstetric interventions and serves to challenge the usual rhetoric of clinical objectivity. These anxieties were articulated explicitly by one medical interviewee: 'I don't want to impose on the husband my sex' (1982: 112).

The ultimate sanction, which was at the time used not uncommonly, comprised the suggestion that the baby's welfare might be threatened by the father's presence. The rather questionable logic featured the possibility of staff failing to resuscitate a baby in a poor condition due to the staff's perception of pressure from the father. A more accurate scenario consists of, when the obstetrician is 'in trouble'; his unease due both to the clinical situation and the father's presence might adversely affect his efficient functioning. Hence it may be that it is defensiveness which is the crucially decisive factor.

Many of the medical misgivings about the father's presence in the labour room are thrown into sharp relief by Brown's discussion of the opposition to his being present in the operating theatre for a caesarean operation. Of course the 'infection' argument is raised, albeit typically unconvincingly. More authentic is what was termed the 'psychology' of the operating theatre. By this is meant the lewd remarks about the 'patient' which serve to promote the much sought-after medical objectivity by distancing the medical staff from their unconscious client. Similarly, teaching opportunities would be seriously curtailed by the father's presence. Interestingly, and a point which will be revisited, is that Brown found that the presence of the father was regarded as acceptable if the caesarean was being performed under epidural anaesthesia (see Chapter 8, p. 167).

Brown concludes, optimistically, that the satisfactory presence of the father in the labour room would be facilitated by a more appropriate birthing environment. It remains to be seen whether the gradually improving labour room environment has been associated with the anticipated change for the father.

Childbirth being changed

The introduction and the, albeit limited, acceptance of the father into the labour room is but one of a raft of changes in the care of the woman in labour which occurred during the latter half of the twentieth century. It may be that the establishment of the National Health Service (NHS) in 1948 and the associated escalation in the proportion of hospital births underpinned many of the subsequent developments in the provision of maternity services (Stephens, 1998). These developments would have had the effect of removing from the father any vestige of a role in labour and childbirth, such as that which he retained when home was the usual place for birth to happen. Although not widely recognised as such, the late twentieth-century changes in maternity care in the UK mirror in many ways the events which occurred during the mid- to late nineteenth century.

The twentieth-century move of childbirth into maternity hospitals may be seen to correspond with the widespread opening of 'charitable' institutions in Victorian times. These institutions included infirmaries, asylums and (for childbearing women) lying-in hospitals. Whereas the earlier events were purported to be philanthropically based, their twentieth-century equivalents are able to claim only NHS policy. In both scenarios the 'patient' regarded herself as the recipient of superior – that is, medical – treatment. The sub-plot was the need to locate and bring together patients who were 'interesting cases' to serve as teaching material for medical students. In the nineteenth century, patients who were insufficiently 'interesting', such as those with infections or degenerative conditions, were not admitted; hence, they found themselves at the mercy of the Poor Law system, that is, in the workhouse.

Late twentieth-century maternity care may be seen to resonate with the events of a century earlier in that large numbers of childbearing women provided suitable 'material', not only for teaching medical students and training grades, but also for medical research. In this way, and on both occasions, the twin aims of consolidating medical power and establishing obstetric professional status were achieved by the implementation of one strategy (Oakley, 1989: 216).

The twentieth-century phenomenon that is maternity care has been based on the medical model and has resulted in the medicalisation of childbearing. Stephens (1998) lists a series of interventions which constitute examples of this process. These include the routinisation of interventions such as continuous electronic fetal monitoring, prophylactic episiotomy and ultra-sonography and, of course, the increasing use of the caesarean operation. She emphasises that these interventions were introduced without the benefit of evaluative or any other forms of research, which is definitely a further point of comparison with the events of the nineteenth century.

A form of intervention which Stephens omits from her list, but the effects of which may be even more insidious and wide ranging, is active management of labour. Again, the twentieth-century augmentation of labour has much in common with the use of ergot and obstetric forceps by the nineteenth-century man-midwives. Active management is the brainchild of a series of 'Masters' of the National Maternity Hospital in Dublin, Ireland. The original rationale was claimed to be pity on the part of the Master for the suffering of women enduring the rigours of prolonged labour, although a high birth rate in a country with limited health provision has also been cited as another reason.

Active management is characterised principally by close monitoring of the woman's progress in labour by frequent – that is, literally quarter-hourly – vaginal examinations. If the rate of cervical dilatation fails to stay above the 'action line' on the partograph, then intervention is indicated, in the form of artificial rupture of membranes and an intravenous oxytocic infusion. The Dublin regime presents a picture of a form of management of labour which verges on the 'military efficiency' to which the authors have referred (O'Driscoll and Meagher, 1986: 89). Active management, though, features the dominance of the partograph to determine the timing and extent of inter-ventions to augment or accelerate labour. This form of monitoring in labour has been appropriately described as 'neo-Taylorist ' after 'Speedy Taylor', who was one of the twentieth century's less humane occupational psycho-logists (Mason, 2000: 247). This approach has been imitated in many industrialised, as well as less developed, countries with questionably beneficial results for the woman and her baby.

The process of the medicalisation of childbirth is recounted by Kitzinger (2000) in terms of the development of risk perception. Risk avoidance and the existence of an 'as if' or 'just in case' mode of management (see Chapter

2, pp. 44–5) is sufficient for risk to become a self-fulfilling prophecy. Kitzinger's words resonate with those of Oakley (1989) who analysed the relationship between the masculine profession of obstetrics, science and maternity services. Oakley identifies the conflict between the masculine form of knowledge, which serves as the basis of obstetrics, and the more feminine forms on which midwifery knowledge and skills have traditionally been founded. The obstetrician's knowledge is supposedly derived from science and the implementation of systematic research-based knowledge. Oakley extends this background into the Cartesian view of the female body as a mere machine which needs the control or the 'mastery' (1989: 217) of a medical practitioner to achieve physiological functioning.

The emphasis on 'mastery' in Oakley's work deliberately reflects the socialisation of men to assume control over all that is near to them, by which she means 'their own fates, families and environments' (1989: 217). Oakley recognises the inevitability that this mastery had, eventually, to be extended to assume control over birth.

This assumption of control over the birth happened in spite of, or perhaps because of, the traditional and historical foundation of the care of child-bearing women with women midwives. The emergence of midwifery, unlike other forms of care, has always been a function of the community within which the childbearing woman lived. Thus the basis of midwifery is social, in which women cared for each other at times of need, such as labour and birth. The women with more experience of providing such care became recognised among their peers as holding special expertise. As Oakley correctly states, 'midwives must do everything to retain this concept of care' (1989: 219). Cahill builds on Oakley's ideas to suggest that the stereotypical assumptions about women which underpin obstetric practice 'compromise and disempower' childbearing women (2001: 340).

The foundations of the obstetrician's scientific credentials, however, are not all that they may seem. If science is taken to mean 'knowledge based on systematic research' (Macdonald, 1981), obstetric practice falls far short of scientific practice, as scathingly observed by Cochrane (1972). In response to Cochrane's biting criticism of his obstetric colleagues, the edifice which is evidence-based medicine has grown up. In spite of this, many of the interventions which Stephens (1998) lists have become and continue to be routine practices in spite of convincing evidence that they improve neither fetal nor maternal outcomes.

Common ground

Oakley's argument about the role of medical men in bringing about changed childbirth may appear to be irrelevant to the father. In spite of this, I am suggesting in this section that there may be commonalities in the approaches of the two groups to the childbirth experience. It may even be possible to suggest that the two groups of men may have fostered or facilitated each other's progress.

Aspirations and assumptions

The foundations of this argument may be found in certain shared views which emerged in the research undertaken by Jackson (1984). He interviewed one hundred men who were in the process of becoming a father for the first time. Each man was interviewed on two occasions: once immediately before and once shortly after the birth. In the research findings this group of men make it very clear who their reference group is and with whom they feel themselves able to identify during their partner's labour. The reference group is the one that the men refer to as 'doctors'. This occupational group features prominently, to the virtual exclusion of any other personnel providing care in labour. An example is one father who reported on the birth of their child being assisted with obstetric forceps. During the forceps birth, the medical practitioner allowed some blood to splash on to his partner's forehead. The father's surprise emerges loud and clear in the father's report of when: 'The doctor actually wiped it away himself and said 'sorry' (1984: 74). The fathers may, of course, have been responding to the labour ward hierarchy and seeking to ally themselves with the most powerful group. This valuation of medical status emerged in one father's explanation of the benefits of giving birth in the hospital setting: 'All them doctors – in case there's any bother' (1984: 81). This statement, as well as demonstrating the man's unalloyed faith in medical infallibility, indicates the assumption of the pathological nature of childbearing. Such assumptions are a well-recognised and fundamental feature of the medical model of childbearing. Thus these assumptions are common to the two groups of men. As well as these issues, it is necessary to question whether a shared gender, or gender orientation, may also be an encouraging factor. Any assumptions of status or shared gender appear to have been valued, with the father 'growing' in the direction of his role model. This involved the father assuming some of the attributes of the medical staff, such as distance, objectivity and authority: 'I kept telling her [what she had to do]. I felt a bit like a doctor' (1984: 67).

It is necessary to question whether such aspirations, assumptions and behaviour are likely to have any effect on the father's relationships with his family. It may be that these factors would reduce any likelihood of the father being able to share his partner's experience of the birth or to initiate his relationship with their baby.

The problem of pain

The experience of pain is fundamental to childbirth. The nature of labour pain, however, is unique in that it has been described as a 'positive' or 'productive' pain (Kitzinger, 1989). It is the healthy or physiological nature of this pain and the outcome – the birth – which differentiates labour from other forms of pain. This crucial differentiation appears to be lost on some, including those who have not or perhaps never will experience labour pain. This lack of differentiation is supported and endorsed by the medical mind-set which is unable to distinguish labour pain from other pathological forms of pain. In this mind-set all pain is inevitably regarded as part of a disease process and, as a result, requires total elimination through medical intervention.

In the same way as the father regards the medical practitioner as his reference group, the father adopts the medical mind-set with regard to pain. This mind-set is aggravated in the father by two factors that are inherent in the situation in which the father finds himself. The first of these factors is the man's close and loving relationship with the woman experiencing the pain. Because of the paternalistic society in which we live, this loving relationship inevitably carries with it an element of protection of the woman, which verges on the assumption of responsibility for her well-being. This 'loving responsibility' means that the man finds difficulty witnessing the distress being experienced by his partner due to her labour pain.

The second factor which is another commonality between the medical mind-set in the father's is, again, a feature of the society to which we belong. This factor is not unrelated to the one already mentioned. It is the assumption among men that they are invariably able to correct, remedy or remove the problems which they or those close to them face. The realisation soon dawns on the father that he is not actually able to remove his partner's pain. This means that he is effectively impotent in this respect, which makes his self-esteem and presence even more difficult to sustain (Johnson, 2002a).

This challenging situation in which the man finds himself becomes apparent in a quote used on the National Childbirth Trust website:

> One thing I felt able to help with was to help Judie use gas and air during contractions. I feel competent with machines, so this felt like something I could contribute.
> (http: //www.nctpregnancyandbabycare.com/article.asp?article=98)

This doubly problematic scenario is supported by the findings of a survey of fathers attending childbirth education sessions (Nolan, 1994). This survey adopted a sympathetic approach to the father and the difficulties which he encounters when accompanying his partner in labour. His experience is appropriately summarised and entitled as 'a journey into a woman's world' (Nolan, 1994: 25). The questionnaire was completed by thirty fathers who were attending National Childbirth Trust antenatal classes. Of particular interest in the present context are the views which emerged on the men's concerns about childbearing. The concerns about the labour included general aspects, such as the man's anxiety about getting the woman to the hospital in time for the birth and the problem of 'coping with the unknown'.

More significantly here, pain features prominently in these men's worries. For 30 per cent of the fathers (n = 9) the 'suffering of the partner' caused them concern (Nolan, 1994: 27). Forty-six per cent of the men (n = 14) were doubtful of their own coping ability, and were asking themselves 'How will I cope with her pain?' Thus even during pregnancy the dual problems mentioned above were making themselves felt. On the basis of these responses, Nolan drew conclusions similar to those outlined above. She concluded that the man experiences a range of fears about his ability to cope with his partner's labour. These fears are centred around his anxiety about his losing control during her labour when, as a man, he is ordinarily in control of events.

The father's apprehension about pain manifested itself further in Nolan's data on the father's unsatisfied informational needs. The men identified a number of areas in which they felt their knowledge was lacking. This suggested that the men perceived more knowledge as the answer to their anxieties, rather than learning coping strategies or practical techniques. In this part of her questionnaire Nolan drew up a rating scale of the topics about which information was sought. The notional maximum for the scale was 300. The topic which scored highest, and which demonstrates both the men's anxiety and the narrowness of their focus, was 'Drugs for pain relief'. This topic scored 242 out of 300 (ibid.).

Thus it appears that his attitude to pain is crucially significant to the father's expectations of his role during childbirth. Further, the 'double whammy' in which I suggest that the father finds himself is supported by the research literature.

Risk and coping

Yet another area in which the father and the medical practitioner have been said to share a common view of childbearing is in the risk involved and the strategies used to cope with that risk.

The risk reduction strategy espoused, but not necessarily practised, by medical practitioners is evidence-based medicine. In his highly respected work on evidence-based care, Walsh (2000a, 2000b) examines the benefits to the woman and baby of two practices which feature prominently in medicalised birth. After reviewing the literature on the assessment of progress in labour, he condemns the routine interventions to accelerate or augment labour on the grounds of their iatrogenic effects. Such effects are most easily measurable in terms of the rising caesarean rate. A more disconcerting measure, though, is the emotional trauma which may be caused to the woman by repeated, and often unnecessary, vaginal examinations. Walsh blames such suffering for postnatal post-traumatic stress disorder, and links it to the woman having been sexually abused.

The limited benefits of medicalisation to the baby follow on from Walsh's (2000b) review of the literature on electronic fetal monitoring (EFM). He clearly demonstrates the immense and authoritative literature base indicating the lack of neonatal benefits in the routine use of EFM. Walsh appropriately goes on to show the risk, in the form of maternal and neonatal morbidity, which is commonly associated with the usual intervention in response to a dubious EFM trace; that is, caesarean. The maternal morbidity of caesarean features both short-term and long-term problems with physical health, while the emotional relationship between the mother and child is thought to be jeopardised.

These issues of risk arise in the report of her study of men in the labour ward by Brown (1982), who contemplates the relevance of the medical model. She concludes that the medical model defines even the relatively uncomplicated birth as a risky event. For this reason medical practitioners attempt to reduce the risk by transforming the birth into a medical event through a panoply of interventions. It stands to reason and is obvious to all concerned, according to Brown (1982: 110), that the father has no place at a medical event. If the birth were a social event, then the situation would be entirely different, but that is not how it has been defined by the most powerful occupational group.

Thus Brown regards the father's presence as being quite incongruent. The only way that the father is able to reduce his incongruity is to effectively camouflage himself, so that he merges in with the medical background and is able to pass unnoticed. The father is able to make his presence less obtrusive by the adoption of a certain coping strategy. This strategy comprises his assumption of the behaviour and attitudes of the dominant medical group (Brown, 1982: 110). This argument resonates powerfully with the findings and conclusion of Jackson (1984).

The general principles of maternity care – that is, medicalisation – have been shown to exemplify the alliance between the father and the medical personnel. Further, I have shown that this alliance is likely to operate to the detriment of the woman. There is, though, another, more specific, example. As mentioned above (pp. 93–5), the problem of pain in labour presents the father with a particularly acute set of challenges. The father's difficulties may be easily resolved by a pain control intervention such as epidural analgesia. Interestingly, it has been suggested that this form of pain control may also bestow certain benefits on the occupational group that provides this service (Mander, 1993, 1994a). Again, the risks to the woman of this form of pain control have attracted relatively limited research attention and publicity (Howell and Chalmers, 1992).

Conclusion: the 'unholy alliance'

In this chapter I have attempted to analyse critically the roles of the male actors when the woman is in labour. It has been shown, both anecdotally and through research, that the father encounters some difficulty in coping with the uncertainties which are inevitably inherent, even in uncomplicated childbirth. Research into the woman's perspective suggests that his difficulty and ensuing anxiety are all too clearly apparent to her. As a result, her awareness of his discomfort constitutes an additional burden for her at a time when she needs all of her energies to be concentrated on giving birth. The uncertainties with which the father has difficulty coping are manifold. They include uncertainty about, first, the outcome of the labour in terms of the health of the woman and baby. Second are the uncertainties relating to the duration of labour, which appear to be challenging. The third and greatest uncertainties have been shown to be those arising out of the father's misgivings about his partner's labour pain. These misgivings relate to not only the severity of the pain, but also to the father's difficulty in coping with his inability to remedy the pain.

Through the medicalisation of childbearing, the obstetrician has sought to resolve his uncertainties about the unknown outcome, duration and pain of labour. The changes contributing to medicalisation to ensure better outcomes have featured greater surveillance. This applies both to the maternal condition, in the form of checking progress in labour, and to the fetal condition, through the increased use of continuous electronic fetal monitoring. The duration of labour has been manipulated through the use of the partograph, which is inseparable from the interventions to augment or accelerate labour, using the principles of active management, which it requires. Such interventions carry with them an increased likelihood of other procedures to terminate the labour, such as the caesarean operation for 'failure to progress'. The active management of labour has brought with it a greater need for pharmacological methods of pain control. This has been associated with the increasing availability of methods such as epidural analgesia. These changes have been introduced in spite of the possibility of such methods actually increasing the necessity for further interventions to counteract their iatrogenic or unwelcome side effects (Howell and Chalmers, 1992).

I have suggested in this chapter that the interventions which constitute the medicalisation of labour may be perceived by the father as a form of uncertainty or risk reduction. Thus the father, an impotent witness to a process which is alien to him, perceives medical personnel as intervening to 'rescue' his partner from what he regards as being a disconcertingly worrisome situation. In this way and for these reasons the father welcomes the obstetrician, for undertaking the role which he, because of his all-too-obvious limitations, is prevented from performing. As noted by Mold and Stein (1986), some obstetricians recognise the medical need to be seen to be doing *something* for or to the woman in labour, even though that something may have no beneficial effect for either the woman or her baby. The benefits, I suggest, accrue to the obstetrician, who is fulfilling his medical role, and the father, whose inability to remedy the situation is excused, if only by proxy. Thus the father finds a welcome and like-minded ally in the medical practitioner. Similarly, the obstetrician welcomes the support he finds in the person who is supposedly the woman's closest collaborator, which allows, or even encourages, him to practise an increasingly interventive form of maternity care.

It is necessary to question in whose interests this alliance operates. The interests of the father are clearly served in terms of the reduction of his uncertainty and, hence, his anxiety. The interests of the obstetrician are served to the extent that his interventive practice is endorsed by those considered to be the consumers of maternity care. The extent to which the woman and her baby benefit from such interventive practice, though, is quite a different matter (Fraser *et al.*, 2002; Howarth and Botha, 2002).

These general and specific examples provide evidence to underpin the argument being advanced here. The argument is that the mutually supportive, even dependent, alliance between the father and the obstetrician during labour is not necessarily to the benefit of the woman who is in labour. For this reason, I venture to suggest that it may be quite appropriately entitled an 'unholy alliance'.

> She (partner) wanted it natural . . . all she kept saying in the run up to going in to hospital was 'No drugs! No Drugs!'. . . . The pain was bad at one point and they said it was time for her to 'stop being stubborn' and have drugs . . . I had them (midwife/medical staff) at me to talk her 'round, and I had promised her (partner) I wouldn't let them . . . the thing was I could see both sides and I didn't know what to do.
>
> (Johnson, 2002a: 175)

Chapter 5

The reality of fatherhood after the birth

Introduction

In Western society the criticism has long been levelled that the father in domestic situations may be regarded as a mere adjunct to the mother. This supplementary status is likely to be viewed unfavourably when compared with the ideal of him enjoying his own unique relationship with their children (Bedford and Johnson, 1988). In this chapter I aim to show that this general observation has been identified to no less an extent by researchers who investigate the development of the new family.

In order to begin to develop this argument I will first examine the research on certain fundamental activities which are crucial to the provision of care in the new family. I will then move on to consider the implications of these activities for the man who is becoming a father. The concepts addressed in this chapter will manifest a progressive shift in their level of abstraction. By this, I mean that I will begin by focusing on essentially practical aspects of family functioning. I will then move through to higher, less concrete levels of interaction, until the realm of the father's self-perception of his own functioning is reached and addressed.

The terminology encountered in the fatherhood literature to which I refer is fraught with dangers. The man who is in the process of becoming a father may be termed a 'new father'. This is problematical because it does not indicate whether or not he has been a father before or whether he has the aspirations to involvement which may be associated with the so-called 'new man'. For these reasons I avoid the term 'new fatherhood' and hope to avoid the uncertainties encountered in the otherwise admirable work of Barclay and Lupton (1999). I will rely on using phrases such as 'first-time father', 'becoming a father' and 'involved fatherhood' in order to prevent such confusion from arising.

As with most work on fatherhood, the research findings referred to in this chapter should be interpreted with some degree of caution. This is due to the widely recognised and accepted difficulties of obtaining research access to a suitable sample of men and of recruiting and retaining that sample (Smith,

1995: 19). It should not be surprising, therefore, that much of the research on the father's behaviour relies on the reports provided by his woman partner. This phenomenon may relate to the woman's stereotypically greater accessibility and willingness to speak to researchers. Hence there is a need for caution. Without intending to mislead the researcher, the woman partner may be providing information about other menfolk she has known, or wishes she had known, rather than providing unbiased factual information.

This chapter may need to have a health warning attached to it. This is because the man who generously agreed to read it argued vehemently that the research literature had been seriously misinterpreted and, as a result, the chapter is quite wrong. He was genuinely concerned, until he happened to discuss the material with the exclusively female secretarial staff. Then a different view emerged.

Practical matters

The father's input into domestic and baby care activities is a topic which tends to generate more heat than light. Reports of his increasing input may be assumed to be a reflection of couples' changing attitudes towards the father's role. Whether this assumption is valid will emerge in the course of this chapter. I would like in this section, though, simply to examine some of the research evidence on the reality of the father's contribution.

The opening statement to this chapter, that the father may be regarded as a mere adjunct to the mother, is supported by the early work of Hill (1987). He found that the father might feign distaste for or incompetence in the less appealing baby care tasks: 'I never got (nappy changing) right – it would fall down, so I'd just have to leave him' (Mr Villiers, in Hill, 1987: 210). This 'incompetence' might be endorsed by the mother, who might require unrealistically high standards of her partner. The same task might be unappealing for reasons of delicacy, even to men in socially challenging work: 'I've not got a very strong stomach. Wet ones, yes, but the other ones, no' (Mr Johnstone, in Hill, 1987: 212); 'My stomach doesna' take it' (Mr Baxter, in Hill, 1987: 212).

As part of a large study based in Avon, England, Smith (1995) examined a range of late twentieth-century data sources to assess the changes over time of the father's involvement in baby care tasks. As well as other sources, a modified snowball technique was used to recruit the women informants. The number of women for each decade varied from ninety-nine who gave birth in the 1950s, to sixty-nine from the 1970s to 286 whose babies were born in the early 1990s. The groups of mothers who gave birth earlier were first asked whether they had any help with baby care tasks and, if so, who provided that help. Each mother was then asked specifically whether her husband or partner assisted with infant care. The examples which were provided, by way of prompts for the women, included bathing, feeding, walking and settling the baby down for the night. Interestingly, it was only the women in the 1990/91 sample who were asked 'how often' the partner undertook these tasks. For the other women there is no indication of the regularity or frequency of the partner's contribution. The data appear to record merely that he had undertaken the task in question. Obviously, this may mean that the father in question had done it as rarely as on only one occasion.

Not surprisingly, Smith found an increase in the reports of the father's input. This upwards trend was not a smooth progression, though. In the 1950s group 39 per cent of women reported some input by the father. In the 1960s and 1970s this had risen to around 55 per cent. By the 1980s and 1990s the reports had risen to around 90 per cent.

Smith highlights bathing the baby as a good example of changing behaviour and, possibly, attitudes. She maintains that during the 1950s, there was a common assumption that the man was not *physically able* to bath the baby. This was associated with fears that he would possibly harm the baby to the extent of causing her death by drowning. Smith's contemporaneous study, however, suggests that in 1995 this was the most popular task for the father, with 75 per cent of men reported to have bathed their babies. As mentioned above, though, there is no indication of the frequency of the man's performance of this activity.

Smith goes on to compare the rising trend of the mother's employment outside the home with the perception of increasing paternal involvement with practical care of the baby (1995: 24). While the trends clearly correspond, Smith is at pains to establish that maternal employment does not *cause* greater paternal involvement. She leaves the reader wondering whether, even if not causative, there may be other common factors involved in this association.

Smith's findings of the father's increasing involvement in baby care serve to support and build on a large and more authoritative study which was undertaken by Brannen and Moss (1988). These researchers examined the functions undertaken by new mothers returning to work after maternity leave. The study showed that the burden of responsibility for domestic and child care arrangements still remains firmly in the hands of the mother. Thus, her routine responsibilities were shown to include the holding down of her full-time job, the arranging for and monitoring of infant care, as well as the completion of most of the household chores. In addition, these researchers show that non-routine activities, such as ensuring effective child care when the usual arrangements break down or caring for the baby when she becomes ill, invariably fall to the woman rather than to her partner (Brannen and Moss, 1988: 158–9).

Building on these studies in England, the work undertaken by Ranson (2001) in Calgary, Alberta is significant in a number of ways. It is particularly valuable for the light which it sheds on the culturally prominent image of the 'new father' (2000: 3). Ranson's was a qualitative study involving twenty-two married men who were engineering graduates. These men were prosperous. Only seven of the men's wives worked outside the home and, of these, only two worked full time. The age of the children ranged from 3 months to 6 years. The men were asked about the relationship between their working life and their family life.

It may be assumed that the 'new father', if he exists, would be easily identified among this group of well-educated and economically secure professionals. Ranson found, however, that the work-focused, breadwinner role still predominated. His family responsibilities were permitted to 'intrude on and reframe' (2000: 22) this role to only a very limited extent. Among these men, the conventional 9 to 5 eight-hour day was widely regarded as a minimum obligation. An equally prevalent finding was the men's assumption that their woman partners (even when they were employed) would be available to take over any family commitments if the demands of his work unexpectedly got in the way of arrangements. Thus, in these highly significant aspects, the men's working lives are shown by Ranson to assume a priority over both their family lives and their partners' working lives.

On the basis of these research and other findings it is clear that, even though roles are perceived as changing, the change falls some way short of any degree of equity in the sharing of parental responsibility. In their work on masculinities, though, Hawkins and colleagues (1995) advance the argument that the issue of equity in parenting is not of prime concern. They accept that the father's underinvolvement in family activities has been established as a fact of life. Further, they recognise that the existence of such under-involvement leads to an imbalance in the parental relationship and, potentially, to conflict.

These authors attempt to reframe the issue of the father's participation in child care. They do this by focusing on the positive developmental aspects of child care; that is, the concept of 'generativity' developed by Erikson (1963). Hawkins and colleagues argue that the father is deprived of, even excluded from, this developmental phase through the mother's intimate and enduring involvement with their child. In this way, they argue, the mother continues her maturation at the expense of the baby's father, who remains relatively underdeveloped. The answer, they suggest, is more help for the father in his acceptance of parental responsibilities.

The patently obvious fallacy of this argument lies in the assumption that child care is invariably and only a pleasurable experience. They ignore the hard work, anxiety and frustration which may occasionally manifest themselves alongside the unalloyed delights of parenthood. This omission, I suggest, renders their thesis untenable.

These equity-related ideas are developed further by Kurz (1997: 96), who draws attention to the difference between the household chores and the infant care tasks which the parents allocate to themselves and to each other. It is usual for the mother to take on the 'low control' tasks which are largely responsive, have tight deadlines and, hence, generate higher levels of stress. Such tasks include the preparation of meals and feeding and shopping for groceries. These tasks may be contrasted with the 'high control' tasks, which would include household and car repairs, and which are less stressful. This is because they are occasional tasks, which do not involve deadlines and are able to be completed at the discretion, perhaps even leisure, of the person doing them.

Breast-feeding

It may be that most of the baby care activities mentioned above represent those which are commonly required by all babies. They are the types of behaviour which are relatively neutral and uncontentious, being able to be performed by a range of carers, including the father. In modern Western society, though, breast-feeding is fundamentally different.

This difference is, first, because the possibility of anybody other than the mother breast feeding a baby is unlikely to be even mentioned. Exceptions to this observation may be found in the work of Storr (2003) and in Lunn (2002). In spite of the almost entirely maternal input to breast-feeding, a range of other family members may also be peripherally involved. Of particular interest is the father's contribution, which has attracted considerable attention among researchers and others (see below).

Second, breast-feeding may be regarded as different because some people will consider that there is some degree of choice about whether or not a baby is breast-fed. While a baby who is not bathed is unlikely to suffer serious consequences, baby bathing is relatively uncontentious and is undertaken with little thought to the costs or benefits. The life-threatening problems arising from a baby not being breast-fed are, on the other hand, well documented (Wilson *et al.*, 1998). In spite of this, there still exists a widespread perception of there being a choice in this matter to the extent of the playing field sometimes being regarded as level.

The male partner or father of the baby is likely to be able to contribute to breast-feeding at a number of points. The first of these is at the time of the breast-feeding decision.

The breast-feeding decision

The work of Ann Thomson (1989) was an early but important contribution to our understanding of the importance of the father's role in this context. This researcher undertook a series of semi-structured interviews with sixty-six first-time mothers during pregnancy and the postnatal period. Of particular interest was the woman's discussion of her feeding method and the influence of family and friends on her infant feeding decision. Thomson found that the woman's mother and partner were the people with whom she was most likely to discuss feeding. The data show that 74 per cent (n = 49) of women discussed the method of feeding with the baby's father and, of these, 71.4 per cent (n = 35) of women decided to breast-feed. Of the 55 per cent (n = 36) women who discussed the feeding method with their own mother, only 58.3 per cent (n = 21) decided to breast-feed. Thus, on the basis of these data it appears that the influence of the prospective father is considerable and is likely to be in favour of breast-feeding.

More recently in Cleveland, Ohio, an anonymous survey was applied to the mothers of one-day-old babies. The aim was to identify factors which would affect the mother's decision to breast-feed (Littman *et al.*, 1994). Unlike Thomson's longitudinal prospective study of the developing decision, these researchers relied on a one-shot survey to generate data relating to the woman's feeding intentions. Because the survey was distributed only in a relatively small private maternity unit, the sample comprised only middle-class white women. The survey sought information on the woman's infant feeding plans and her intended duration of breast-feeding. These feeding outcomes were correlated with the woman's report of, first, the father's attitude to breast-feeding and, second, the feeding practice of her female relatives. The response rate was high at 74 per cent (115 responses out of 155 questionnaires distributed).

Littman and colleagues found a strongly significant correlation between father's enthusiastic approval of breast-feeding, his higher level of education and plans for the baby to be totally breast-fed ($p < 0.001$). Although these findings may be interpreted as showing the benefits of the father's contribution to the infant feeding decision, caution may be necessary in their interpretation. This is mainly due to the homogeneity of the sample. Caution is also necessary because, as so often happens, the mother's reports were used to attempt to measure the father's attitude.

A large survey was undertaken in Perth, Western Australia, which sought information on the mother's attitudes and beliefs about breast-feeding and the influence of her significant others on the infant feeding decision (Scott *et al.*, 1997). The mothers were recruited in two maternity units within three days after the birth and a self-administered questionnaire was applied. Fifty-eight per cent (n = 556) of the 948 eligible women completed the question-naire. The women were asked about the preference of the baby's father and whether the mother's mother had breast-fed at least two children. While education, family income and the partner's occupation were also influential, the father's feeding preference was most significant. Scott and colleagues found that women who perceived that the father preferred breast-feeding were ten times more likely to initiate breast-feeding. On this basis, these researchers conclude that the father's preference is the most important factor.

The rationale for the woman deciding not to breast-feed was the focus of a study in England (Earle, 2000). This research is relevant here due to the prominence the women attached to ensuring that the father was able to take advantage of the opportunities presented by formula feeding to relate to their child. The father's involvement in feeding was perceived by some mothers as a form of 'time out' for her in which she could be relieved of some of the less welcome obligations of motherhood. These mothers regarded breast-feeding as not permitting such relief. While this relief was just that for some of the mothers, for other women it became no more than an opportunity to catch up with the multiplicity of other tasks awaiting their attention. Thus it may be that breast-feeding would be more likely to provide the relief which the mother was seeking.

On the basis of these studies in the UK, USA and Australia, it appears that the woman who perceives her partner as supportive of her intention to breast-feed is more likely to decide that that is how she will feed her baby. Further, although these data are more limited, she appears to go on to implement that decision. It could be that the woman's perception of being supported in her initiation of breast-feeding is likely to make her more confident in the early difficult days. This perception of support may augur well for the accomplishment of her plans. The studies mentioned thus far, though, have not sought to find out from the father how he views the issue of the infant feeding decision.

This omission has been addressed to some extent by the North American research of Freed and colleagues (1992). These researchers recruited a sample of men who attended a childbirth education session. Although childbirth education in the USA attracts a broader spectrum of men than its UK equivalent, the male respondents in this study were, according to the authors, not representative of the total population, being 'better medically informed' than others (1992: 225). This criticism of the unrepresentativeness of the sample is supported by the ethnic mix, which was overwhelmingly white. The researchers do admit this limitation, however, when they state that their results reflect a 'best case scenario' (ibid.).

Clearly the sample surveyed by Freed and colleagues was, yet again, slightly unusual. In view of this bias, it is interesting to note the attitudes to the woman, her body and her feeding practices which were held by the men in the sample. Over 20 per cent of the fathers expecting their child to be fed a breast milk substitute agreed that breast-feeding is not natural and that the woman who is breast-feeding is less attractive. Around 50 per cent of these men agreed that breast-feeding is bad for the breasts and that it makes the breasts ugly. A large proportion of all of the fathers agreed that breast-feeding interferes with sex; the figure for the fathers of formula-fed babies was 75 per cent. Of the fathers whose babies were to have breast or mixed feeding, almost 40 per cent in each group agreed with this statement. It is apparent that, even in this relatively educated and affluent sample, pro-prietorial attitudes to the woman and her body may influence the woman's health behaviour.

These attitudes were brought home forcibly to me on one occasion recently when I was attending a couple in the labour ward. Ella had just given birth and Steve was staying with her. I asked her if she would like to breast-feed her new baby. Before Ella had a chance to open her mouth, Steve replied for her: 'She's nae getting her tits oot on top o' the bus.'

The reality of breast-feeding

The research literature on the father and the practice of breast-feeding has traditionally presented a uniformly bleak picture. The way in which this picture has emerged is traced in this section.

The early and most highly influential research on the role of the father during breast-feeding was undertaken in Seattle, USA (Jordan and Wall, 1990). In the course of a large study of the man's experience of pregnancy and parenthood, these researchers 'serendipitously' (1990: 210) illuminated his experience during breast-feeding. Grounded theory methodology was used, involving a mixed sample of fifty-six men, half of whom were interviewed six or seven times around the time of the birth. The father's enthusiasm for his child to be breast-fed was clearly apparent from the interviews during pregnancy. Each father was found to anticipate a role which involved 'essential maternal nurturing' (1990: 211). Jordan and Wall imply the shock of the reality of breast-feeding in terms of the man being surprised to find himself excluded from the woman's relationship with their baby. This was found to be comparable with the way in which he had, shortly before, been excluded from her relationship with the fetus.

The recognition of the cultural significance of food and feeding is raised by Jordan and Wall in relation to the father's need to do *something* for his child. If the baby was one of those who refuses to take a feed from a bottle, the father's overwhelming feelings of inadequacy were cruelly reinforced. This happened to some fathers in spite of the parents' plans to give the baby a bottle on a regular basis in order to facilitate the father's relationship with the baby. These researchers report that the father was required to use his entire repertoire of tactics, or 'bag of tricks' (1990: 211), to console or try to satisfy his child. His partner, by way of contrast, needed only to hold the baby for the calming action of the promise of impending nourishment to take effect. The need for the father to be able to feed his child was found to be crucially important to these men. When the baby complied, the man would be able to feed her using a bottle. For the father of the non-compliant baby, however, he was obliged to wait until the child was ready for solid foods to be introduced, before establishing his relationship with her.

In terms of the father's relationship with his baby, Jordan and Wall found that the father was required to work hard in order to identify and develop unique facets of the relationship. For many of the fathers, though, breast-feeding was a time during which he was compelled to take a 'back seat' (1990:

211). This terminology resonates with the experience of men attending childbirth education (Smith, 1999b, 1999c; see also Chapter 3, pp. 73–5 above). That the back seat was not a comfortable position to adopt emerged in the words of one father who spoke of 'sacrificing' his relationship with his child (Jordan and Wall, 1990: 211). His sacrifice was continued for the duration of breast-feeding, in anticipation that he would be able to take up the relationship when the child was weaned.

The fact that these data emerged serendipitously may cast doubt on their validity. The importance of breast-feeding arising as an issue during pregnancy is not entirely clear. This is because Jordan and Wall state that each father was confident of the future and would have perceived no need to discuss breast-feeding. It was only when the man started to realise that breast-feeding was beginning to be a problem that he and the researchers would have had to begin to focus any attention on it. In this way the pregnancy data should really have been disregarded, and the 'shock' effect dismissed as an artefact. These data would only have been of value if breast-feeding had been the major focus of the research from the outset.

In compliance with the tenets of the practice of grounded theory, Jordan and Wall follow the presentation of their data by a comparison with the extant literature. This proved problematical in view of the lack of research attention to the father's role. When his role does appear in the literature it is only the one involving support for the lactating mother which is highlighted. On the basis of these findings, Jordan and Wall argue that both parents should be prepared more realistically for their role. It is inevitable that this preparation would present a picture of a decidedly dismal experience which would have the potential to become a self-fulfilling prophecy. It may be that this is an example of the 'negative advertising' to which breast-feeding has always been vulnerable. This form of advertising is one which is used widely to promote a product, such as a breast milk substitute, not by showing its value but by discrediting its competitors (Watson and Mander, 1995).

Jordan and Wall's ground-breaking work has much in common with a slightly later study by Gamble and Morse (1993). Both of these studies are North American, though on different sides of the border. Both used grounded theory methodology and both succeeded in interviewing the father, rather than relying on the mother's report. It may not be surprising, therefore, that there are some commonalities between the findings. The bleak picture of the father's experience presented by Jordan and Wall, however, is moderated somewhat by the findings of Gamble and Morse.

The perception of exclusion from the mother–child relationship encountered by the fathers in the Jordan and Wall study was modified in the Gamble and Morse study to 'postponing' the relationship. This involved the father of the breast-fed baby delaying or putting on hold his formation of his relationship with the child. This was achieved through his gradually increasing awareness of his limited role and his eventual acceptance of that role. The father was able to identify some factors which reinforced his acceptance of this, to him, less than satisfactory arrangement. These are factors which are consistent with his high expectations prior to the birth, such as the 'neat' nature of breast-feeding (1993: 361). Other factors were identified which served to compensate him for his relinquishment of the anticipated relationship. These factors were the other activities which did not involve breast-feeding. The postponement eventually ended and the father was then able to 'catch up' with the formation of the relationship.

The research by Gamble and Morse, as well as illuminating the father's less than satisfactory experience, demonstrated an important aspect of the father's functioning. It may be assumed that, because the mother and the father are generally regarded as carrying out fundamentally different roles in the reproductive process, they would recognise them as different. Gamble and Morse, however, suggest that this is not the case. They found that the father is not aware of or does not accept these crucial, probably anatomical and physiological, differences. These authors write: 'These men were touched by the nature of the mother–infant relationship and used this as a standard against which to measure their own relationships with their infants' (1993: 359).

It may be that such expectations should be regarded as foolish and that failure is inevitable when such a high standard is applied. The question which arises, though, is whether the father is prepared to face such a scenario. Perhaps his socialisation, the pressure on him to be involved and the assumptions of equity lead him to expect an equitable balance of involvement in the relationship stakes. Careful thought, however, soon leads to the realisation that such comparisons are doomed to failure.

Thus it is apparent that Gamble and Morse, while presenting a generally more optimistic picture of the father's experience, have drawn attention to one particular area with profound and irrevocable implications. These disconcerting findings resonate with those found in a very different UK study. In their work on the thorny perennial problem of promoting breast-feeding among disadvantaged women, Whelan and Lupton (1998) happened upon the limited role of the partner in this situation. The researchers note the small number of men who pressured their partners to discontinue breast-feeding. They surmise that this is probably due to the women with unsupportive partners having been unlikely to even begin breast-feeding and so be excluded from the study. Whelan and Lupton found that the partners were most likely to be found 'taking a back seat' (1998: 97) in the same way as the father in Jordan and Wall's study did. The woman found that this approach to breast-feeding was distinctly unsupportive and was replicated in the emotional and practical support which the man provided. For these reasons the woman resorted to the help and support of other women, especially her own mother.

A more recent Canadian study seeks to apply a rather different 'spin' to the existing picture of the father's experience of the mother breast-feeding their baby. The work of Storr (2003) is, like Jordan and Wall (1990) and Gamble and Morse (1993), North American in origin. Like them she undertook a qualitative study, but hers was based on a phenomenological, rather than a grounded theory, methodology. The volunteer fathers were relatively affluent, as may be expected when they were recruited mainly through childbirth education. Unlike the other two North American studies, though, each of the fathers who Storr interviewed repeatedly through the perinatal period did seem to have found a role for himself. Rather than regretting his lack of any input, the father in Storr's study was able to, in his view, make himself indispensable to the success of breast-feeding. She summarises this phenomenon as 'nurturing their partners so they can nourish their babies' (2003: iv). In this way the father is able to maintain his relationship with his partner as well as both directly and indirectly relating to their new infant.

Providing support

The challenges of the postnatal period have for too long been ignored in favour of images of idyllically happy mothers and contented babies. In this idealised scenario the father has been assumed to do little more than keep out of the way. Research is now being undertaken and has been published which suggests that the reality may be different.

An example is a largely qualitative study of social support in the postnatal period which was undertaken in England using feminist research methodology (Podkolinski, 1998). It examined the postnatal experiences of ten women, each of whom lived with a male partner, who together with the baby's grandmother provided most of the support. The woman experienced intensive support from these sources for a period ranging from six to seventeen days. This researcher identified that practical support, in the form of helping with household tasks, is as important as emotional support. The partner's support was found to vary in the extent to which it met the woman's expectations. Podkolinski gives examples of partners who were thought to expect too much of the new mother. 'Julie' is one example who, at four weeks, was still having difficulty breast-feeding to the point of her baby not having regained his birth weight. Her partner could not understand why she could not leave their son with a babysitter in order to go to the pictures with him. 'Julie' went on to write in her diary: 'I think that more information should be thrust at men, as Bret does not seem to understand what I'm feeling. It's all I can do to wash up the breakfast dishes each day' (Podkolinski, 1998: 220).

Podkolinski's findings resonate with the data which emerged from Gamble and Morse's (1993) grounded theory study of the father of a breast-fed baby (see pp. 107–8 above). Their data permitted a typology of fathering styles to be drawn up which derived from each man's account of his activities, and which appear to illuminate his supportive role. The researchers related these activities to his previous role, his work/education and his assumptions about the nature of fathering.

Gamble and Morse were able to identify four fathering styles which clearly indicate the support which he was or was not able to offer his partner:

- The *involved* father who believes in and seeks to practise equity in decision-making and household/child care activities.
- The *'assistor'* father who tends to be supportive and encouraging rather than taking an equal part. Because this father is limited in his child-related activities, he tends to resort to DIY tasks to demonstrate his need to contribute. He is keen to relate to the baby, but tends to be relegated to her playtime.
- The *supervisor* father has definite ideas about child care, but his activities are limited to the 'clean and dry' baby (1993: 363). This father is likely to be relieved that his involvement with other aspects of child care is minimal.
- The *detached* father does not have strong feelings about baby care or about his contribution to it. This father is likely to perceive his role as being more related to activities outwith the family home.

Although these four fathering styles may appear to be stereotypes, this may not be the case. The authoritative research which identified them should encourage acceptance of their existence. This typology and its impression of partner support should be kept in mind while considering other aspects of becoming a father.

Becoming a father

As well as his supportive role, a wide range of other aspects of the experience of becoming a father were addressed in a survey organised by the National Childbirth Trust (NCT). The usual problem of gaining access to and retaining a sample of men faced the researchers Singh and Newburn (2000). A possible solution to this problem was found in the database of the 'sampling organisation' Bounty UK Ltd (Bounty, 2003; Watson and Mander, 1995). Through this database the researchers were able to access each of the eligible women to request that the questionnaire be passed on to her partner. The limited success of reaching a sample of men in this way is evident from the poor response rate of 37 per cent. Out of 2,300 questionnaires distributed and followed up with reminders, there were only 817 (35.5 per cent) which provided usable information.

The men who did respond, though, gave a wide-ranging picture of embarking on fatherhood. For some of the men, the experience was one of unmitigated pleasure: 'Every day she does something new. It's a constant source of joy. I love every thing about her' (First-time father in sales, in Singh and Newburn, 2000: 65). The researchers, however, ultimately had to conclude that: 'at the very least, men tend to find life with a new baby challenging' (ibid.).

Singh and Newburn observed that the men who already had children were better able to take becoming a father in their stride. First-time fathers found the experience 'overwhelming, worrying and scary' (ibid.), although this was just what they had said they expected when they had completed their antenatal questionnaires.

This study found that, in the event, the men's main concerns were not markedly dissimilar from those of their female partners. Not surprisingly, 'tiredness' featured prominently, being a major problem for 17 per cent of the men and a minor problem for a further 37 per cent. Very close behind tiredness in a scale of the father's most common concerns came 'starting sex/painful sex'. This was reported to be a major concern for 12 per cent of the men and a minor concern for a further 28 per cent.

Probably more importantly, in order to obtain a good understanding of the experience of the father, the father's impressions of the baby's behaviour appear to speak volumes. The men were generally happy with the baby's sleeping pattern: 'His sleeping pattern doesn't affect me. I do not wake up' (First-time father, journalist, in Singh and Newburn, 2000: 66). 'I feel OK about his sleeping because my partner deals with night feeds, as I work and need my sleep' (First-time father, petrol station worker, in ibid.).

Singh and Newburn consider that their data support others' observations that the father has 'fewer difficulties getting enough sleep' (ibid.). They go on to report, by way of examples, some more of the comments which led them to their view:

> It is OK now but at first it was a real nightmare. It didn't affect me that much but my wife was up and down all the time to feed him.
>
> (First-time father unemployed, in ibid.)

> To be honest, although I feel tired sometimes, it mainly is my girlfriend who deals with all the crying at night and changing nappies and feeding. I go to work in the morning and she stays at home so I need my sleep more than her.
>
> (First-time father, semi-skilled worker, in ibid.)

The man's experience of becoming a father begins to emerge clearly from the admittedly small, and possibly unrepresentative, sample accessed by these researchers.

In this chapter I have moved from the most practical aspects of becoming a father in the direction of the less tangible areas. The work of Woollett and Parr (1997) clearly illuminates the more emotional challenges for the man facing fatherhood. These challenges include not only those involving his relationship with the new baby, but also those in which his relationship with his partner are involved. These researchers obtained a high (76 per cent, n = 106) response rate to their longitudinal study by recruiting couples through women attending an antenatal clinic. The attrition rate was only 5 per cent in the series of questionnaires and interviews. Interestingly, though, these losses were due to couples splitting up and/or the man being unwilling to respond.

The men in Woollett and Parr's study invariably scored higher – that is, more positively – than their partners in their feelings about pregnancy and the early and late postnatal period. The researchers suggest that, in spite of the rhetoric of 'sharing and paternal involvement' (1997: 180), this positive orientation is associated with the birth of the child impinging on the man's life to a far lesser extent than on that of his female partner. They go so far as to suggest that 'there is little evidence that most fathers are substantially involved' (ibid.). Thus first-time parenthood, they argue, is not likely to have the potentially life changing effect on the man that it has on the woman. This is attributed in part to the man assuming the traditional breadwinner role, and thus limiting his activities in the home. The relationship and activities with the baby are recognised by Woollett and Parr as rapidly becoming the focus for the couple. This means that their former pre-occupation with each other is suddenly and quite unexpectedly displaced. These researchers suggest that this unexpected displacement is the major reason for the tensions which they found commonly arise within the couple's relationship after the birth.

Like Woollett and Parr in the English home counties, Barclay and Lupton (1999) focused on first-time fathers, but in Australia. This latter study was totally qualitative, using discourse analysis, and quite appropriately involved only fifteen men. The time period for the two studies was similar, extending from pre-labour to about six months later. Barclay and Lupton's study serves to re-emphasise many of the issues which have been raised above. This authoritative study not only establishes that the issues have existed, in case of doubt, but also indicates that they continue to exist.

There is one important issue in the Barclay and Lupton work, which resonates powerfully with some of the quotes from Singh and Newburn (2000: see p. 111 above). This is the man's attitude to work, meaning his distinction between his own paid employment as breadwinner and the woman's activities involving household tasks and child care. This distinction involves the man's prioritisation of his employment. It is she who is required to attend to the baby at night since, he seems to assume, she is able to catch up on her sleep during the day. It appears to be difficult for the man to imagine that caring for a small child is anything other than undemanding.

The expectations of each of the men who Barclay and Lupton interviewed emerge as being of tremendous importance. These expectations included fashionable jargon such as 'bonding' and 'being there', which the researchers sought to unravel. These terms, though, had very little generally accepted meaning; they were associated more with what might be termed the man's 'unfinished business' in relation to his own father. This means that the man is merely reacting against his own experience of being parented. Thus a knee-jerk reaction is happening in which he is seeking to ensure that his child's experience is different from his own.

The man's expectations of newborn infant behaviour were shown to be, to say the least, not quite realistic. Barclay and Lupton found that the man was surprised by the baby's 'unexpected immaturity' (1999: 1019). This resulted in the man being somewhat uncertain about his role. As one father explained: 'There is not much I can do. You can't really get her on a bike and go for a ride at this stage in her life' (1999: 1016).

As well as the man's uncertain expectations about his own functioning with the child, there were found to be other problematical expectations. These refer partly to the man's expectations of the woman's work within the house, in that it was not his role. There were also, though, her expectations of herself, by which are meant her ability relative to his incompetence. It may be that tensions were aggravated through even the low-status women's work in the house being denied him.

In the same way as Gamble and Morse (1993; see pp. 107–8 above) found that the man compares his functioning and relationship with the baby with that of his partner, Barclay and Lupton identified a similar phenomenon. The Australian study found that the man perceived that by breast-feeding, the woman is 'privileged' (1999: 1019) in her close and nourishing relationship with the baby. Barclay and Lupton repeatedly describe the man as 'resenting' or 'being resentful of' (ibid.) the woman's privileged status in this respect.

Like Woollett and Parr (1997), Barclay and Lupton recognise the tensions that are likely to arise within the couple's relationship after it reaches its idyllic peak at the time of the birth. By way of contrast, the relationship is under greatest stress around the second or third week after the birth. This is when the woman is finding that her support systems are rapidly falling away and the man has returned to his employment. Both are making demands of the other which are perceived as excessive. Barclay and Lupton consider that a shared expectation of structure to their family life is crucial. This may be a shared need for a highly structured life, as in the example of a couple who were born-again Christians. Alternatively, the shared need for a highly unstructured life worked in the example of a very young couple who both realised that they had a lot to learn about becoming parents.

Unlike other researchers mentioned above, the men in Barclay and Lupton's sample found becoming a father infinitely more 'disappointing and frustrating' (1999: 1019) than they had expected. As in the Gamble and Morse sample, the men were forced to accept that they would have to occupy a position relegated to the fringes of parenthood for the first six months of the child's life. On the basis of this large and authoritative study, these researchers present a bleak impression of the experience of becoming a father at the end of the twentieth century. They go on to report that, even though the media and some men would argue to the contrary, in the context of fatherhood, the 'new age man' was found by their research not to exist. It may be suggested that the society in which this research was undertaken may not be conducive to such male aspirations. The fact, however, that Barclay and Lupton's work resonates strongly with other countries' research indicates that this is not actually the case.

Intrapersonal abilities

In this chapter I began with some contemplation of the more practical aspects of fatherhood and have moved to focus on the most abstract. In order to examine these, I use the term 'intrapersonal' abilities, which represent a range of characteristics which combine to contribute to emotional intelligence (Bar-On, 1997; Goleman, 1996). These characteristics are closely linked with a 'developmental perspective' to the process of becoming a father (Hawkins et al., 1995). These authors' definition of this perspective incorporates an adaptive ability which facilitates the move from simpler to more complex skills, such as child care. This definition is next expanded to include characteristics which resonate with intrapersonal ones, such as perceptions of one's own status and functioning as well as others'. It is clear that this perspective is likely to be helpful in understanding the experience of the man going through the process of becoming a father.

One of the theories of human development which tends to underpin much current thinking about personality and which contributes to the 'developmental perspective' is the one advanced by Erikson (1963). While his major focus was on childhood and adolescent development, Erikson gave some attention to adult tasks and others have subsequently built on his ideas. Of particular importance has been the task which he labelled 'generativity', which features the need to learn to care for others. This concept was elaborated in Erikson (1982), which related this form of care to the need to guide the next generation in order to ensure its firm grounding. The nurturing of the person's own offspring serves to achieve this altruistic ideal by ensuring a suitable environment in which subsequent generations are able to progress. Erikson assumed a holistic orientation in the search for this ideal, so it is not limited by family or by society or even by generation. He considered that a failure to achieve generativity carries with it the risk of stagnation to the extent of interpersonal impoverishment.

The concept of generativity, Erikson maintained, was important not only to the future of the human race as a whole, but also to the individual who does or does not achieve this state. He regarded generativity as a fundamental characteristic of the fully mature human being. Rather disconcertingly, this form of maturity has been interpreted as being available to a man only if and when he becomes a father (Hawkins *et al.*, 1995). In spite of such decidedly questionable assumptions and statements, there appears to be some reluctance to question or criticise Eriksonian theory. Particularly perplexing is the rigid nature of his theory of human development. This theory makes allowance for 'crises' of identity only at given points, while at other times requiring 'commitment' to the chosen identity (Waterman, 1999: 594). Little allowance appears to be provided for the dynamic processes that are fundamental to development. The dynamic process of becoming a father is a good example in view of the multiplicity of uncertainties which, as I have already shown by reference to research, tend to beset him. In spite of this unnecessarily rigid framework, Hawkins and colleagues (1995) use Eriksonian theory to argue that the solution to the modern problems of fatherhood lies in encouraging the father to assume greater responsibility in child care. This, they suggest, would also correct the mismatch or dissonance between the developmental stages of the two parents associated with differing experiences. In this way, they argue, the threat of conflict in the couple's relationship would be able to be reduced.

The role of parenting as a crucial stimulus to adult development was the focus of a study by Palkovitz and colleagues (2001). These researchers also relied heavily on the work of Erikson in planning their qualitative study of forty fathers in the Eastern USA. Perhaps not surprisingly, each of the men maintained that the arrival of a child had been a crucial factor in his maturation as a man. This maturation involved certain themes: 'settling down', 'becoming less self-centred', 'accepting major responsibilities', 'experiencing generativity' and 'fatherhood as a jolt'. The difference which fatherhood stimulated was considered by one man to have been extreme enough to turn him away from a life of crime. While the authors emphasise that the men really believed that it was becoming a father which had made all the difference to each of the men, they admit that this is not possible to confirm objectively. The views of the women who were the mothers of the children might have provided valuable corroborating data. Similarly, the voices of the 'children' themselves would have been a welcome contribution to these men's stories. The research cited above indicates that the views of these significant others may differ from those of the father.

A study based mainly in Montreal, Canada, resolved some of the questions left unanswered by Palkowitz and colleagues. In their transcultural work with Canadian and Japanese couples, Steinberg and colleagues (2000) studied the birth and postnatal experience. This study showed the changing meaning of the term 'fatherhood' to the various participants with the passage of time, indicating its dynamic nature. As has been mentioned elsewhere (see Chapter 3, p. 64), the lack of a role model is a problem for the father. This results in him, as was noted above (Barclay and Lupton, 1999), needing to deal merely with his own 'unfinished business' when becoming a father. Steinberg and colleagues, like Barclay and Lupton (1999), also identified the domestic difficulties faced by the couple in the postnatal period. They found that the couples endured 'dyadic conflicts' (2000: 1270) during their attempts to renegotiate the organisation of mundane household tasks.

In terms of the psychosocial development of each of the parents, Steinberg and colleagues identified important differences. These researchers found that the 'developmental trajectories' (2000: 1270) were prone to diverge vastly, with traumatic consequences. This observation resonates with that of Hawkins and colleagues (1995) as mentioned above, in that the woman's development is likely to be kick-started by the unavoidable intensity of her experience of motherhood. The father, on the other hand, has the option of adopting a very traditional role which may leave his maturational development largely unaffected. Steinberg and colleagues recommend that the woman should be able to act as a mentor to her partner in his maturational development and in his attempts to contribute to household and child care tasks. Such a recommendation appears to ignore the possibility that it would give the woman a further burden with which to cope. Further, this would be happening at a time when efforts should be being made to ameliorate her challenging situation, rather than aggravate it.

This developmental orientation also emerged out of a phenomenological study of the father's experience by Deane-Gray (2001). This midwife researcher used a psychoanalytical orientation to scrutinise the father's involvement in the birth in particular. She identified the man's involvement as a 'rite of passage'. Rather than being a transition to manhood, as such rites usually are, this 'rite of passage' initiates the man into fatherhood.

Conclusion

In this chapter a picture has been presented of the experience of the father after the birth of the baby and how this experience may affect the process of his becoming a father to the new baby. The difficulties facing the man and the couple have emerged clearly from the research findings. The extent to which they are or are not able to help each other has also emerged.

The role of the father as merely adjunctive to the mother has been addressed. The literature suggests that this situation pertains in many developed cultures. There is also a prevalent belief that this arrangement is less than ideal to the various actors who participate in the drama which is the establishment of a young family. One difficulty which appears to be well established is the problem of the chronicity of the father's experience and the potential for a long-term effect on his relationship with the child. Two major studies have identified problems in this area. Barclay and Lupton (1999) found that the father was required to take a back seat in the early days of infancy. Similarly, Gamble and Morse (1993) found that the father considered that he had to 'postpone' the assumption of fatherhood. The concern which these findings leave is that the man may be missing out on his big opportunity. It could be that by the time the circumstances are ready it will be too late to establish the relationship with the child which he seeks. This is because the family relationships will have become too firmly entrenched to permit change.

The difficulties which face the new father were summarised for me in the following terms:

> It is a sad irony that on the one hand men are told of the importance of fatherhood and the necessity for active fatherhood if children are to be happy and healthy.
>
> Problems such as crime, drugs and abuse are all attributed to failed or absent fathers. If this is not enough to guarantee paranoia, it is hard to tell what is.
>
> Yet, [on the other hand] the maternity system and social expectations all conspire to render the job and the expectations of the new father at best unrealistic and at worst impossible.
>
> (Jacobs, 2003)

Chapter 6

Childbearing and domestic violence

Introduction

The relevance of a chapter on domestic violence to a book on men and childbearing may require a certain amount of explanation. This is supported by my personal experience of talking to colleagues, students and lay people about domestic violence and childbearing in preparation for this chapter. The need for an explanation also mirrors the observation by Bewley (2002a) of the attitudes of senior midwifery personnel and obstetricians in 1990. She identified: 'disbelief and reluctance to accept domestic violence as an issue for health professionals' (Bewley, 2002a: S3). This 'disbelief and reluctance' is not, however, unique to senior maternity care staff. It is my personal and recent observation that a secretary's broken jaw, associated with her partner's football team having lost its game, was a source of considerable hilarity in a gathering of (mainly male) academics.

In spite of such dismissive attitudes, to a disconcertingly large number of women the connection between domestic violence and childbearing needs no explanation whatsoever. It is possible that this may be because they belong to the group of women for whom childbearing is invariably and in-extricably linked with the violent behaviour of the father of the baby or of a previous partner. The reader for whom the connection needs to be explained is likely to be fortunate enough not to have had this personal experience. This is not to suggest that only the woman who has experienced domestic violence is able to make this connection or to empathise with the woman who is abused. This is certainly not the case. As with so many aspects of care, personal experience is not necessary for it to be effective. Knowledge and understanding of the abused woman's wish to be listened to and believed are without doubt more significant (Bewley, 2002b).

In this chapter I demonstrate the significance of the phenomenon which is often known as domestic violence and its importance in childbearing. I do this by, first of all, examining the terminology which is used and the various meanings. Second, the characteristics of domestic violence in child-bearing are addressed in terms of the nature and size of the problem, then the underlying factors and the implications. Third, an attempt is made to outline the interventions which have been recommended and how these recommendations impinge on the role of the midwife and others who provide care for the childbearing woman. The conclusion draws together the issues raised in the chapter in order to show the reader the significance of this material to an understanding of men's involvement in childbearing and maternity care.

Definitions, terms and meanings

The problem which is often known as domestic violence has only really been recognised as such since the mid-twentieth century (Pizzey, 1974). This recognition reflects a painfully slow change in societal attitudes from the days when the only limitation on the male partner's behaviour was the diameter of the instrument which he could use to inflict 'punishment'. It was in this way that the 'rule of thumb' came into existence, based as it was on the maximum diameter of the rod which a man was permitted to use to chastise his wife. The extent of the change in societal attitudes is addressed below in the section on the nature of the problem.

Pizzey's original term, 'wife battering', soon proved to be too unacceptable for general use. This was due not only to its graphic nature, but also to its lack of precision. The woman involved may not actually be in or have been in a marital relationship with her abuser. This point is highly pertinent in view of the possibility that it is the threat of the ending of any relationship that may have triggered the abuse (Mezey, 1997a: 37). Further, the term 'wife battering' is not appropriate because it serves to limit the form of the violence visited on the woman. In fact, the forms which the violence takes appear to be infinite (Lloyd, 1997).

In addition, the word 'domestic', as in domestic violence or domestic abuse, is less than appropriate for two reasons. The first is that the term suggests a degree of domesticity or family conviviality which certainly does not apply in the abusive relationship. The second is that 'domestic' implies that the problem is small scale or insignificant which, again, does not apply. Lloyd (1997) links this latter point with a widespread underestimation of the gravity of the problem. She maintains that by the use of such terms domestic violence is 'trivialised' (1997: 5), which carries the implication that it is not sufficiently serious to make it worthy of public concern. Thus this form of abuse is permitted to remain a private, family matter. Further, it is deprived of the serious attention from policy-makers which it urgently needs and deserves.

The North American term 'intimate partner violence' (McFarlane et al., 2000), while quite precise and suitably explicit, carries the disadvantage of being rather unwieldy. For these reasons and because some form of violation is fundamental to this phenomenon, the terms 'domestic violence' and 'domestic abuse', though less than satisfactory, will be used synony-mously here.

In order to define domestic violence, it is necessary to take account of a range of factors which have been shown to be associated with it. First, the relationship which is the context of the violence is crucial, although it may be either ongoing, ending or over and done with. The sexual nature of the past or ongoing relationship is of fundamental importance. Second, the abuser's behaviour obviously matters, but in view of its variability, attempts to define it are probably futile. Similarly, to distinguish between the woman's feelings of violation and the man's violent acts (Lloyd, 1997) is pointless in view of the interdependence of these phenomena. The balance of power between the abuser and the subject is clear and indisputable, although the situation may be more complex than it at first appears. Finally, Lloyd raises the distinction sometimes mentioned between the deserving and the undeserving victim. She correctly dismisses such a distinction as a form of victim blaming, worthy only of being discounted. Before doing so, however, she indicates that such dangerous attitudes are by no means unknown among some sections of society and even within the criminal justice system.

Lloyd goes on to question whose definition of domestic violence is the most appropriate. Bearing in mind the exceedingly slow grinding of the wheels of the criminal justice system, the legal definition is at risk of being hopelessly out of date. The professional definition, however, may reflect the narrow gender, social class and ethnic background of the professions' members. Lloyd suggests that the definition produced by women is the one which may be the most useful, an example of which was developed in a large and authoritative research project which is discussed below (Mooney, 2000).

For the purposes of this chapter, the definition used is one drawn up by women. It features in the website of a national charity which addresses domestic violence perpetrated against a range of vulnerable subjects. This definition is particularly useful in that it clearly indicates the broad-ranging and long-term nature of the problem:

> Domestic violence is physical, psychological, sexual or financial violence that takes place within an intimate or family-type relationship and forms a pattern of coercive and controlling behaviour.
>
> (Women's Aid, 2001)

Appropriately, the major focus in this chapter and more generally is on the violence which men visit on their women partners and ex-partners. In comparison, the trauma experienced by men at the hands of their women partners has been identified as 'marginal' (Bewley and Gibbs, 2000: 101). This problem of 'woman on man' violence has probably attracted more publicity and research attention than it really deserves (Dobash et al., 2000). An example of such research is the work of Migliaccio (2002), which found that the factors underlying this form of violence correspond in many ways with the indisputably more prevalent 'man on woman' form. Violence within same-sex relationships is also the subject of somewhat less research interest (Cruz and Firestone, 1998).

The nature of the problem

As summarised in the definition offered above, domestic violence may assume an almost infinite number of physical and non-physical forms. On the basis of her large and authoritative North London Domestic Violence Survey, Mooney (2000) provides a comprehensive picture of domestic violence in a mixed community. This three-stage study involved 571 women and 429 men, representing a response rate of 83 per cent from the 1,205 households approached.

The women in the sample defined domestic violence in terms of the following five behaviours:

- *Mental cruelty* – verbal abuse/ridiculing, sleep deprivation, money, clothes, liberty
- *Threats* – of physical force or violence
- *Actual physical violence* – hitting, pushing, shaking, kicking, head-butting without actual injury
- Physical injury – bruising, black eyes, broken bones
- Rape – sexual intercourse without consent.

The level of agreement among women respondents for each of these statements was high, at 68 per cent to 92 per cent. Mooney was able to assess the frequency with which each of these forms of domestic violence was experienced by the women respondents during their lifetimes (Table 6.1). On the basis of these data Mooney is able to draw the conclusion that a quarter to one-third of women have been subjected to domestic violence at some time during their lives.

Table 6.1 The prevalence of domestic violence in women's lives by type of violence (n = 430)

Violent behaviours	%
Mental cruelty	37
Threats	27
Actual physical violence	32
Physical injury	27
Rape	23

Source: Mooney (2000: 155)

Domestic violence during childbearing

It might be assumed that pregnancy may serve to protect the woman from the abuse of her partner. This has been shown by research evidence to be far from the case (Scobie and McGuire, 1999). In fact, the reverse is more likely to be so. The incidence of domestic violence associated with childbearing is significant and, in addition, it demonstrates certain characteristic features.

The nature of domestic violence during childbearing

It is well recognised that domestic violence during the childbearing cycle is usually associated with a number of characteristic injuries. Mezey (1997b) suggests that, typically, the site of the injury at this time is likely to be related to the woman's reproductive functions. This means that the woman is more vulnerable to injuries to her breasts, to her genitalia and to her perineal area. Additionally, a particularly likely site for her to be attacked is in the region of her pregnant abdomen, as shown in Table 6.2. The latter trauma may result in damage and wounds, not just to the woman, but also during pregnancy to the fetus. Because these are the parts of her body that are ordinarily concealed by clothing, Scobie and McGuire (1999) argue that she may be able to hide the physical evidence of her abuse. They go on to suggest that this form of deception involves some degree of collusion by other family members who are aware of the abusive relationship. If the midwife chooses not to act on the injuries which the privileged nature of her contact reveals to her, this means that she is also effectively colluding in the woman's abuse.

In a large study, recently completed in England by Mezey and Bewley (2000), 892 childbearing women were screened for domestic violence. Of the twenty-two women who had been subjected to domestic abuse during their current pregnancy, data were obtained on the site of the woman's injuries in nineteen cases (see Table 6.2).

Table 6.2 Site of injury following domestic abuse during current pregnancy (multiple responses were recorded)

Site	Number	%
Face	10	56.2
Abdomen	7	36.8
Head	5	26.3
Back	4	21.1
Wrists	3	15.8
Breasts	3	15.8
Arms	2	10.5
Legs	2	10.5
Fingers	1	5.3
Shoulders	1	5.3
Neck	1	5.3

Source: Mezey and Bewley (2000)

These data provide limited support to the general impression of the woman's 'reproductive' organs being vulnerable. The variably serious nature of the injuries arising out of these assaults on childbearing women is apparent from the data presented in Table 6.3.

Table 6.3 The type of injury sustained due to domestic violence (multiple responses were recorded)

Injuries	Number	%
No lasting pain/injury	5	23.8
Persistent pain	4	19.0
Cuts and/or bruises	9	42.9
Injury needing hospital treatment	4	19.0
Permanent disfigurement	1	4.8

Source: Mezey and Bewley (2000: 12)

Closely bound up with the woman's experience of domestic violence are the other forms of harm to which she may subject herself. These harms take the form of her abuse of damaging substances, which she is likely to come to rely on in an effort to cope with her abusive relationship (Bewley and Gibbs, 2001: 183). The inappropriately heavy uses of alcohol and illicit drugs are obvious and frequent examples of such a coping strategy.

One possible result of domestic violence which does not emerge out of the work of either Mooney or Mezey and Bewley is the death of the childbearing woman; that is, a maternal death. This is because these researchers focused on the man's behaviours and the woman's injuries, rather than the outcome in terms of survival. In addition, prior to the ground-breaking work of Mezey and Bewley (2000), researchers had addressed only the problems of women in general, rather than those experienced by women during the childbearing cycle. This omission reinforces the observation by McFarlane and colleagues (1992, 2000) that domestic violence in relation to childbearing is in need of more, as well as more serious, research attention, although this omission may now be beginning to be addressed (Garcia and Davidson, 2002).

Domestic violence as a cause of maternal death was first shown to be a problem in the 'Confidential Enquiries' Report for 1994–96 (CEMD, 1998). The next report in the series (CEMD, 2001) assumed an appropriately greater in-depth approach to the topic, by devoting a chapter to discussing it (Lewis, 2001).

The main purpose of the 'Confidential Enquiries', since they were initiated in England and Wales in 1952 (DoH, 1999), has been not to allocate blame, but to identify areas of care which are amenable to improvement. Thus the aim has always been to prevent further 'avoidable' loss of women's lives. In the most recent Report (CEMD, 2001) the assessors indicate a number of ways in which the maternity services could have better served the eight childbearing women who subsequently died as a result of domestic violence (Lewis, 2001: 241).

The assessors found that, of the 378 women whose deaths they reported, 12 per cent (n = 45) actually volunteered information to a carer about their having been subjected to domestic abuse. This degree of disclosure is exceptional in a woman being abused, as the woman ordinarily avoids such disclosure. This avoidance is because she expects that it would engender further 'punishment' by her abusive partner by way of retribution (Mezey, 1997b: 192). The figure of 12 per cent, however, is unlikely to represent the complete picture, as the standard of care was so low that not one of the 378 women who died had been asked routinely by maternity staff about her experience of domestic violence.

In their report, the assessors found it necessary to criticise communication between carers and women whose first language is not English. The assessors found that, in such situations, independent interpreters tended not to have been called in. This led to the all too familiar scenario of family members, such as partners or sons, acting as translators during the woman's intimate consultations. In addition, the maternity staff failed to recognise or act upon visual and other indicators that the woman was being subjected to domestic violence, such as:

- Late booking and/or poor/non-attendance at the antenatal clinic
- Over-frequent attendance with minor problems or unsupported complaints
- Unexplained admissions to the maternity unit or attendance at the accident and emergency department
- Non-compliance with treatment and discharge against advice
- Minimisation of signs of violence on her body
- Constant presence of the woman's partner and his reluctance ever to leave the woman
- Partner preventing the woman from speaking by answering for her
- Woman reluctant to disagree with her partner.

If the woman was able to report violence to the staff, they offered little or no effective help to the woman (Lewis, 2001: 243).

These data present a clear picture of the childbearing woman being coerced by her abusive partner into compliance. They also show that she was prevented from articulating her situation by his constant presence. The woman whose first language is not English may have been prevented from revealing her abuse by the fact that her abuser may be acting as her interpreter. Alternatively, the interpreter may have been her teenage son or another relative, who colluded in sharing and keeping the family secret. Families were found to have conspired together to keep the fact of domestic violence undisclosed to care providers. When presented with explicit reports and a combination of suspicious signs and behaviours, the staff were not able to intervene effectively to protect the woman and to prevent her death.

In one chapter of the most recent Confidential Enquiries Report, Lewis (2001: 248–50) catalogues a series of cases in which the woman's death was caused or precipitated by domestic violence. These cases comprise a series of vulnerable women. The series includes one woman 'who spoke no English' (2001: 248), one who used intravenous drugs inappropriately, a 'very young schoolgirl' (2001: 249) and a woman who worked in the sex industry. Although the Report certainly does not mention the possibility, there is a question which must be asked. This question is whether each of these women's low standard of care reflected a value judgement on the woman's lifestyle on the part of the maternity staff. A negative answer to this question is only possible in the case of one of these women, whose midwives were found to have acted 'in an exemplary manner' (2001: 247).

The incidence of domestic violence during childbearing

That pregnancy is not a period of respite from domestic violence has been recognised for almost as long as the condition itself has been documented. On the basis of a small study (n = 33), in 1977, Flynn found that 50 per cent of the women in one refuge had been subjected to domestic violence during pregnancy. It may be appropriate to question whether a sample of abused women is a suitable one from which to draw conclusions about the population in general. A similar criticism probably applies to work such as that by Stark and colleagues (1981). These researchers found that 21 per cent of the 2,676 women treated in one accident and emergency department had suffered abuse. They also noted that the women were more likely to be abused when they were pregnant.

The samples used in these two relatively early studies illustrate one of the pitfalls of undertaking research in such a sensitive area. This means that the prevalence of domestic violence in pregnancy is difficult to estimate (Mezey, 1997b: 192). This difficulty is due largely to the woman's reluctance to disclose the situation for fear of the man's violent retaliation. The challenges of conducting research in the area of domestic violence are discussed below (see pp. 132–4).

Some of the problems of sampling and data collection were overcome in the recent study by Mezey and Bewley (2000). Of the 892 childbearing women who were screened on at least one occasion for incidents of domestic violence, 122 women (13.4 per cent) responded positively. Ninety-four women (10.5 per cent) reported having experienced incidents of domestic violence prior to the past year, of whom twenty-nine (3.3 per cent) also reported incidents within the past twelve months.

During the preceding year, fifty-seven (6.4 per cent) of the women screened reported having been subjected to domestic abuse. The researchers, having subdivided the abuse into physical and sexual, found that for a large majority of the women the abuse was physical. A minority of the women (24.6 per cent, n = 14) experienced sexual abuse with or without physical abuse. For both groups of women, those who experienced either or both forms of violence were more likely to be abused repeatedly, rather than infrequently. The frequency of the abuse during the current pregnancy, however, showed a different pattern. More of the abused women reported one incident rather than two or three incidents.

These data clearly reinforce the observation that the childbearing woman is in no way immune from domestic violence. Further, it is widely believed that pregnancy may actually act as a predisposing factor, or a trigger, to domestic abuse (Mooney, 1995; Stark *et al.*, 1981). This is supported by the evidence of the Mezey and Bewley study (2000), as these researchers found that, for seven women in their sample (0.8 per cent), the experience of domestic violence began during pregnancy. Although pregnancy appears to exert the effect on the perpetrators of stimulating violent behaviour, it is during the postnatal period that the woman has been found to be most vulnerable. This was established by a study of the experiences of 275 child-bearing women (Gielen *et al.*, 1994), which involved three interviews during pregnancy and one at six months after the birth. These researchers found that, whereas 19 per cent of the women were subjected to moderate to severe domestic abuse during pregnancy, this figure rose to 25 per cent after the birth. Thus this changing incidence of domestic violence makes it necessary to examine the factors that are believed to underlie this form of abuse.

The underlying factors outside pregnancy

In order to consider the factors which have been suggested as underpinning domestic violence, it may be helpful to consider first the characteristics of the abuser. I will then move on to examine the suggestions which have been made in relation to the predisposing factors.

The perpetrator

In the same way that much antisocial behaviour has been associated with and possibly attributed to personal physical characteristics, the perpetrators of domestic violence have been similarly 'diagnosed'. In her Marxist-feminist analysis of domestic violence, Mooney (2000) traces the historical origins of such positivistic attributions of criminality. She finds that the history of biological positivism is long and undistinguished. In the nineteenth century, criminals began to be regarded as 'throwbacks'. This is because they were seen to demonstrate physical and other features which related to an earlier stage of human evolutionary development (2000: 37). Although Mooney describes how such genetic attributions are currently widely ridiculed, she shows that such ideas still persist among certain groups, such as the evangelical right (2000: 42).

The application of such positivistic ideas to domestic violence served, when its existence was first recognised, to differentiate the abusive partner from the people in society who considered themselves to be 'normal' (2000: 44). This argument has subsequently been refined to 'prove' that domestic abusers, while possibly not actually psychopathological, show at least a predisposition to mental health problems.

Mooney argues that the purpose of such positivistic theories has been to show that domestic violence is a minority activity, which occurs only in the seriously deviant personality. According to this line of thought such behaviour is possible only in a small group of predetermined 'types' who are unable to prevent themselves from indulging in this form of antisocial activity (2000: 44). By criticising this line of reasoning, Mooney effectively demolishes the argument that only a finite proportion of men have the capacity to perpetrate domestic violence against their female partners.

Mooney's feminist analysis of the history of the character of the domestic abuser is supported to some extent by the work of Mezey (1997a). Mental health problems, she maintains in support of Mooney, are rarely a significant factor in the aetiology of domestic violence. To provide further evidence of the premeditated nature of domestic violence, Mezey cites the tactics and strategies used by violent men to avoid recognising their own abusive behaviour. These include the denial, the forgetting and the blanking out of their inappropriately hostile actions (Dobash et al., 2000).

The man's background has been found to be likely to feature seriously low self-esteem, which may be associated with a history of physical and/or mental abuse in childhood. In addition, the man is likely to demonstrate some limitation of his verbal ability, which may have either or both of two serious consequences. The first is that his limited language skills prevent him from talking through his difficulties and, thus, the relationship problems will remain unresolved. The second problem caused by his less than communicative nature arises out of the comparison of his communication ability with his partner's. According to Mezey, this means that if the woman is more articulate and possibly better educated, he will perceive himself to be doubly disadvantaged. In this way the couple's problems will be aggravated further. In such a scenario the woman may threaten to leave the relationship to escape the difficulty. This is likely to exacerbate his violent behaviour, which will escalate due to the increasing threat to the man's inadequate sense of security and need for support. In a situation such as this, however, the man's perception is likely to be less than accurate. This may be seen in that he would give an account of having been provoked to violence by his partner's threat to leave. In their research Dobash and colleagues refer to this form of self-justification as 'blaming the victim' (2000: 33).

In such circumstances the characteristic cycle of violence, first traced by Lenore Walker in 1979, would begin to unfold. The typically cyclical pattern involves the gradual increase in tension within the relationship, followed by the sudden outburst of violence. After the eruption of violence, the man realises the effects of his behaviour and is overtaken and subdued by remorse. In his remorseful state he offers apologies, promises never to repeat the violent behaviour and pledges himself to continuing love.

Predisposing factors

The factors which underpin and precipitate domestic violence range from the virtually universal to the intensely personal. In terms of the broader picture, domestic abuse clearly represents a demonstration of the power of the male partner. The ability of men to subject women to violence is a reflection of the man's physically more powerful build (Mezey, 1997a). Mooney (2000), on the other hand, presents a more incisive analysis of masculine power, by linking it to patriarchal relationships in general and to the capitalist system of political beliefs in particular.

In their midwifery-focused account of domestic violence, Bewley and Gibbs recognise the problem of identifying the causes of a phenomenon which does not even have a 'universally understood definition' (2000: 103). While accepting that this warning appropriately indicates the dangers of attributing causation to a relatively ill-defined phenomenon, it is clear that some discussion of the factors associated with domestic violence is likely to assist our understanding of this form of aggressive behaviour.

The intergenerational transmission of domestic violence has been shown to be an underlying factor by a library-based research project (McClellan and Killeen, 2000). These North American researchers focus on the psychological basis of what they call 'intimate partner violence'. The intergenerational effects, though, differ hugely and fundamentally from the genetic explanations condemned by Mooney (2000, above). McClellan and Killeen draw on the well-known work on mother–infant attachment undertaken by John Bowlby (1958) which used ethological and psychoanalytic principles. Although Bowlby's work has been subjected to widespread, profound and probably justified criticism, his contention that the human newborn attracts loving, caring attention within an affectionate relationship is generally accepted. McClellan and Killeen, however, suggest that if the newborn's relationships with his caregivers are less than reliable, insecure attachments will continue to feature throughout this person's life. These researchers go on to apply attachment theory to 'adult romantic' relationships (2000: 355). The person whose infantile relationships featured insecurity, they argue, encounters difficulty in being confident in the formation of trusting and supportive adult relationships. These unstable relationships are rendered abusive, rather than just unsatisfactory, by certain phenomena which occurred at the same time as the infant was seeking security where none existed. These phenomena account for the intergenerational effect mentioned above. The infant's lack of security may have evolved through an unstable into an abusive personality by either being the recipient of or witness to family violence. The person who is being described by McClellan and Killeen (2000) has been found to demonstrate jealousy, dependency, anger and violence in adult relationships, which may be associated with his long-standing lack of self-respect.

The men who abuse their partners have been shown to protect themselves from the realisation of their violence by projecting the responsibility for it on to their partners. In this way they are able to regard the victim or her behaviour as the predisposing factor. As mentioned above (see pp. 126–8), in this way the abusive man is likely to excuse his aggressive behaviour by blaming the subject of his violence. In their study of an intervention to reduce domestic violence, Dobash and colleagues found that the man would justify his violence by criticising his partner for talking too much or too little, for arguing or not arguing, for being too materialistic or too spiritual, and so on. As well as victim blaming such as this, the man would 'minimise' his violence by underestimating its seriousness and effects. Further minimisation would be achieved by comparing his own violence with the behaviour of other men who are, he supposes, even more violent.

In her assessment of the perpetrator's 'trigger' factors, Stanko raises the problems associated with the abuse of alcohol and other drugs (1997: 20). The complexity of the role of excessive alcohol consumption in domestic violence is addressed by Dobash and colleagues (2000: 29). The disinhibiting effect of alcohol would be the first factor to come to mind, but these researchers also argue that a 'culture' of excessive alcohol intake is likely to provide a fertile environment for violence. At another level, the cost of the man's alcohol consumption may be a continuing source of conflict in a relationship in which financial resources are tight. Another source of conflict may relate to the man's absence if his drinking happens outwith the family home. Thus his absence may be denying the woman the support she seeks with household and family-related tasks.

The relationship between the couple has also been shown to act as the precipitating factor to violence. Dobash and colleagues give examples of the couple's lack of, difficulty with, or disapproval of each others' social lives. The arrival of a new child into the relationship may arouse resentment at the restrictions which she brings, together with conflict over her care and upbringing. As well as featuring as one particular form of domestic violence, sex or its absence may also act as a precipitating factor. Dobash and colleagues suggest that sex is one of the 'services' to be provided by the woman which 'men expect and demand . . . throughout the day and night' (2000: 26). These researchers raise the spectre of marital rape, when one man reports: 'Well, if she'd let me do it [have sex] I wouldn't have punched her.'

Stanko (1997) summarises the trigger factors for domestic violence into four main groups:

1 The man's possessiveness and jealousy may be a source of conflict leading to violence. Anxieties about relations with other men, or former relationships, may threaten the man's confidence in his own relationship. Relationships with female friends and with family have been shown by Dobash and colleagues to engender similar uncertainties.

2 The man's expectations of his partner feature prominently as trigger factors. These may relate to matters such as social functions, to the upbringing of children and to sex. A particularly important area in which expectations may not be met is in the domestic chores or housework. Such household tasks may cause problems by not being done or by not being done to an adequate standard. Alternatively, the house work may be considered to be done too conscientiously or may be done at the 'wrong' time.

3 The man may use violence as punishment for perceived wrongdoing by his partner, irrespective of the reality of the situation.

4 Violence may be used as a prop to bolster the man's authority in circumstances in which he perceives this authority to be under threat. This authority may deny the woman the right to question or debate on the grounds of its nuisance value, as well as its undermining his self-esteem. Dobash and colleagues (2000) regard the man's authority as extending far beyond the verbal arena and into the mundane routines of everyday life, such as finance, child-rearing, property, use of time and mobility outside the family home.

Stanko's four categories of precipitating factors are as likely to apply during pregnancy as at any other time during the woman's life. These four precipitating factors, however, are taken a stage further by Scobie and McGuire who define pregnancy itself as a trigger to bring about domestic violence (1999: 259). This is an issue which certainly merits further serious attention.

The underlying factors during pregnancy

Perhaps not surprisingly, the man who abuses his partner during pregnancy has much in common with the man who abuses her at other times. The difference is that, during pregnancy, another person in the form of the fetus enters the couple's intimate relationship. In addition, the woman interacts with a wide range of other people because of her pregnancy (Helton and Snodgrass, 1987). Both of these factors serve to threaten the limited control which the man is able to exert over his relationship with his partner. This threat is probably the main underlying reason for the increased incidence of domestic abuse during pregnancy.

The man's specific emotional reactions to his partner's pregnancy which result in violence have been recounted by Mezey (1997b). She describes, first, the man's jealousy towards the fetus and baby, on the grounds that the fetus/baby now has an infinitely more intimate relationship with the woman than he does. This is the relationship for which the man himself yearns and of which, in pregnancy and the postnatal period, he regards himself as being deprived. Mezey goes on to describe how the man's jealousy towards the fetus and baby turns to anger when he may actually find himself displaced and inconvenienced. This applies when the woman becomes preoccupied with herself and with the fetus/baby to the disadvantage of the man. His feelings of displacement also manifest themselves when the 'services' to which he is accustomed may be less conveniently forthcoming.

Third is the pregnancy-specific violence which is engendered by the woman's inability to complete some of the functions which he expects of her, and which may be related to her changing body shape. Fourth is the 'business as usual', which includes the reasons for domestic abuse that apply at other times throughout the woman's life.

Mezey goes on to recount the observation mentioned above that during pregnancy not only is the woman at her most vulnerable, but there are also two people who are susceptible to the man's violent behaviour. Thus both the woman and the fetus/baby are at risk of injury and death; the latter possibility gives rise to the spectre of child abuse (Bewley, 2002a). The risks are increased markedly with men who are intravenous drug-users and may lead to homicide and feticide (Mezey, 1997b: 193).

According to Mezey, domestic violence during pregnancy may be envisaged essentially as an attack on the woman's sexuality. Ordinarily the man may be able to control this aspect of her being, but during her pregnancy her sexuality is quite obvious. He may even regard her as flaunting her sexuality, in the form of her changing body shape, for all to see and over which he has no control. Thus the woman's pregnancy may be seen as symbolising her lack of dependence on him. It is clearly something which is seen as hers and part of her so his lack of control is apparent not just to him, but to all.

The abusive male, Mezey argues, endeavours to control his partner's reproduction. This may be through endeavouring to make her pregnant, perhaps by rape, or by avoiding or forbidding the use of contraception. The picture of the domestic abuser as insecure, inadequate and dependent determines his behaviour during pregnancy. His efforts to control his partner are as fervent during pregnancy as at other times, and he seeks to achieve this control by physical and psychological means in order to bind her to him through loyalty, pity, fear or dependence.

It is clear that childbearing alters the balance within the family. This is due primarily to the presence of a/another child who requires her finite resources of attention. Childbearing also brings others into intimate contact with her, including family members as well as professional carers. Such contact increases the risk of the recognition of domestic violence, leading to an increase in the man's insecurity and more violence.

The impact of domestic violence in pregnancy

Domestic violence has long been believed to be associated with a number of adverse effects on the woman's experience of childbearing (Stark *et al.*, 1981). These effects have been shown to apply during the pregnancy and the labour as well as the postnatal period. The recent study by Mezey and Bewley (2000) was able to demonstrate the range of pregnancy complications which are likely to occur more frequently in association with domestic violence (Table 6.4).

Although these researchers found that many of the problems occur more frequently in women who are subjected to domestic abuse, only 'headaches, back pain and hyperemesis' and admission in 'false labour' reached the level of significance.

Mezey and Bewley found no correlation between domestic abuse and 'bad outcomes' to the pregnancy, meaning miscarriage, pre-term labour or stillbirth. In spite of this finding, it is widely believed on the basis of other studies that there is an association (CEMD, 2001: 243; McWilliams and McKiernan, 1993).

The ultimate impact of domestic violence, the death of the mother, has been discussed above (see pp. 123–4).

Table 6.4 Antenatal complications noted during the current pregnancy

Complication	Abuse in past year		No history of abuse		Total (%)	
	% (n = 30)		% (n = 165)		(n = 195)	
Any AN complication	80.6	(25)	66.7	(110)	68.9	(135)
Abdominal pain +/– bleeding	40.0	(12)	24.2	(40)	26.7	(52)
Headache, back pain, hyperemesis*	20.0	(6)	7.3	(12)	9.2	(18)
Unresolved admission	13.3	(4)	5.5	(9)	6.7	(13)
False labour*	36.7	(11)	15.8	(26)	19.0	(37)

Source: Mezey and Bewley (2000)
Note: * Significant at p<0.05

Researching domestic violence in pregnancy

The problem of domestic violence is difficult to resolve, or even to approach, for a number of reasons. Part of the difficulty relates to the secrecy in which it is shrouded. This, as mentioned above, is due largely to a conspiracy of silence within the family. The secrecy is fuelled by the woman's fear of further violence. Together, these phenomena serve to foster the man's denial. Scobie and McGuire support this interpretation when they maintain that domestic abuse 'is still one of the taboos of modern day society' (1999: 259). In their suggestion that the education of the midwife is one way in which the problem can begin to be addressed, these authors implicitly recognise the need for research on which to base such educational strategies. Researching domestic violence, however, is fraught with problems for a number of reasons.

The problem of collecting reliable data has been mentioned above, in the context of relying on the populations of women's refuges. Similar caution needs to be applied when using the figures provided by law enforcement agencies. This is because these agencies are made aware of only a small proportion of all the incidents of domestic violence. Mooney, in further support of such a cautious approach, refers to the 'hidden figure of crime' (2000: 3). By this she means the selectivity of crime reporting, in that not all crimes are reported to the police and that, further, the police may not necessarily record all of the crimes reported to them. The explanation for this mismatch between incidents happening, being reported and being recorded is not easy to assess.

Mooney recounts how 'victimisation surveys' have to some extent illuminated the magnitude of domestic violence. The problem of under-reporting, though, persists, and gives rise to a picture of only the 'tip of the iceberg'. This under-reporting is likely to be due to the fear of inadequate confidentiality for the woman, resulting in anxiety about violent reprisals. Because of the inevitable secrecy surrounding domestic violence, a woman is hardly likely to be able to confide in a totally unknown data collector. With this caution in mind, Mooney quotes victimisation surveys as demonstrating domestic violence rates of between 3 per cent and 8 per cent.

The sensitivity needed on the part of the researcher and data collector to access such personal information should not be underestimated. Suitable training for data collectors incurs heavy financial costs which deplete any research funding. Economies are likely to result in the sample size being reduced, putting the findings at risk of accusations of bias, lack of power and poor generaliseability.

A North American study (McFarlane et al., 2000) shows some of the ways in which researchers have attempted to collect reliable data during a research project on intimate partner violence. These researchers used a face-to-face questionnaire which had been translated into the woman informant's own language; in this way any possibility of her partner being required to act as an interpreter was eliminated. His non-involvement was further assured when all the interviews were held in a private room without the male partner or any other people being present. Unfortunately these researchers do not detail the strategies they used to ensure that the partner was not present. The partner's absence during such questioning is fundamental if it is to elicit reliable information, since the presence of a violent partner would render the woman vulnerable to the threat of retaliation.

The study in England by Mezey and Bewley (2000) attempted to implement similar precautions in order to protect the women informants. The time away from the partner and others during which the midwife, who acted as data collector, could ask about matters such as domestic violence was known as 'confidential time'. Unlike McFarlane and colleagues (2000), who apparently had no difficulty making this arrangement, the midwives were successful in obtaining confidential time with only 40 per cent of the women who were accompanied to their antenatal appointments. These researchers note that persuading the partner to absent himself was also a particular problem during the midwife's postnatal visits to the family home. Such a finding gives rise to considerable concern. This anxiety is aroused by the fact that women during the postnatal period have been shown to be maximally vulnerable to domestic violence (see pp. 125–6 above). Thus the close, continuing and intractable presence of the partner is a source of concern both in practice and in research.

Mezey and Bewley (2000) found that sensitivity to the woman's feelings was not the only precaution necessary in domestic violence research. These researchers appear to have been surprised to find that, in spite of being trained to ask the woman direct questions about domestic violence, many of the midwives found that the emotional costs of acting as data collectors in this study were too great to bear.

Thus the problem of domestic violence in pregnancy is beginning to be addressed by researchers. Despite a coherent and authoritative research programme, though, Garcia and Davidson (2002) recognise that the existing knowledge-base is still 'extremely limited' (2002: S25).

The help available

The strategy prepared by one NHS Trust (Price and Baird, 2001) actually featured consideration of the midwife's ability to cope with the demands of asking questions about abuse. Price and Baird describe how they extended the role of the midwife to include routine screening of the childbearing woman for domestic violence. The midwife's role is crucial in this respect because, as mentioned above (see p. 125), childbearing and domestic violence have a strong relationship. McFarlane and colleagues (2000) take this point further by showing how pregnancy is also a good time for intervention in abusive relationships because of the ongoing contact with potentially helpful care providers. Further, the midwife is clearly in a privileged position in this context. This is because the midwife has access to the woman, in terms of listening to her and observing parts of her body which are ordinarily kept covered. In this way the midwife is in an ideal position to both recognise physical and behavioural signs of abuse and to offer the woman the support and information which she may be seeking.

The strategy described by Price and Baird began with drawing up and agreeing professional guidelines (see Table 6.5). This document provided a foundation for the multi-professional education sessions which targeted different issues and impediments to changing practice. Guidelines such as these allow the midwife to recognise the woman's situation and to give the woman information about the options available to her. The woman is then able to decide what action, if any, she may wish to pursue. These actions may include the location of a place of safety for the woman and her children and referral to Social Services or Social Work departments.

Observations such as that by McFarlane and colleagues (2000) about the possibility of reducing domestic violence by interventions associated with childbearing have resulted in the development of screening tools. A controlled trial in Rhode Island evaluated the use of a screening tool incorporating direct questions (Norton *et al.*, 1995). The sample comprised 234 childbearing women in a relatively deprived area. The researchers found that the detection of domestic violence was significantly higher when the women were asked direct questions. Further, it was found that opportunities for intervention, such as giving information, were created by the use of this tool.

The screening of pregnant women for domestic violence was a major focus of the important study by Mezey and Bewley (2000). These researchers sought to find out whether asking specific and direct questions to screen for domestic violence was acceptable to childbearing women. The results show that asking specific questions is, first, effective in the detection of domestic abuse. Second, these questions were found to be acceptable to women who are abused as well as to those who are not. As mentioned above, though, the toll on the midwife asking the questions proved to be intolerably heavy.

Some examples of questions which have been found to be appropriate include the following:

* Is everything all right at home?
* Is anyone hurting you at home?
* Are you frightened by anyone at home?
* Does your partner break things that belong to you?
* Some women tell me that their partners hit them. Has that happened to you?

(RCM, 1998)

Table 6.5 Principles of professional guidelines

* Recognition of the abuse
* Provision of private environment
* Identification of abuse
* Documentation of abuse
* Provision of information on resources and options.

Source: Price and Baird (2001)

Such seemingly simple questions are intended to help health care providers to break through the barrier created by the conspiracy of silence surrounding domestic violence (Bewley and Gibbs, 2001). In spite of their apparent simplicity, though, these questions need to be used with caution. They should never be asked in the presence of the partner or if a family member is interpreting. Equally, it would be unethical for such questions to be asked in the absence of suitable follow-up. An important systematic review of screening for domestic violence, undertaken by Ramsay and colleagues (2002), endorsed such a cautious approach to screening. On the basis of their review of the twenty papers which met their inclusion criteria, this group of researchers concluded that: 'it would be premature to introduce a screening programme for domestic violence in health care settings' (Ramsay *et al.*, 2002: 26).

These researchers found that, although screening programmes are effective in identifying abuse, the protocols for subsequent interventions to remedy the situation are not yet in place. In this way, the woman's danger would currently be likely to actually be increased by health workers' screening. The research involving all twenty-three consultant-led maternity units in Scotland, however, resulted in slightly different recommendations (Foy *et al.*, 2000). These researchers suggest that a structured form of screening by midwives should be introduced, in spite of their finding of midwives' limited knowledge of sources of support. On the basis of the results of a Swedish study, however, changes to midwifery practice as well as to maternity care policy are suggested (Edin and Högberg, 2002). The Swedish researchers recommend that the midwife should be encouraged to ask direct questions of all of her clients in a suitably private environment.

The input of health care providers is important, for the reasons mentioned above. This input has often been less than helpful, largely because their traditional 'turning a blind eye' to suspicions of abuse effectively condones that abuse (Mezey, 1997a). Bewley and Gibbs spell out the policy implications inherent in encouraging health care providers to address domestic abuse. The acknowledgement of the existence and magnitude of the problem is a first step in providing an appropriate service to women who have been subjected to abuse. The support of 'front-line' staff by the provision of education, guidance and co-operation with other helping agencies is crucial. The involvement of other agencies is a prominent feature of the educational programme organised for midwives and others by Ward and Spence (2002). Although these educators claim to focus on 'screening' for domestic violence, they do not state whether a specific abuse assessment tool is recommended or the 'sensitive questioning' to which Bewley and Gibbs (2001) refer.

The educational programme initiated by Ward and Spence encountered many obstacles, not least the limited funding (2002: S15), which is not at all unknown in work with domestic violence (Bewley, 2002a). This problem, it may be suggested, indicates the continuing low priority attached by policy-makers to this form of abuse. In addition, this problem is aggravated by consideration of the resources spent on other forms of screening for conditions, such as placenta praevia, which show a much lower incidence. The policy-makers' low priority for domestic violence was reflected in the midwives' poor attendance at educational events. The dismal turnout encountered by Ward and Spence may mean that the findings of Scobie and McGuire's study are more representative than these researchers thought. Their small postal survey (n = 67) clearly demonstrated the midwife's reluctance to 'get involved' (1999: 261) with matters such as domestic violence. Such reluctance resonates with the well-recognised professional inclination to 'respect' the woman's privacy when she declines to explain obvious injuries (Mezey, 1997b). Scobie and McGuire blame the midwife's reluctance to get involved on either the fear of inability to do anything or, possibly, the midwife's own painful personal experience of abuse. These researchers, like Bewley (2002a), do suggest that the midwife's attitudes may be the problem, but do not mention that this may be associated with long-standing patriarchal attitudes to domestic violence.

Ward and Spence's educational programme overcame the problems due to lack of funding by 'cascading' the teaching. This involved in-house teaching which made the material more relevant, but meant that the teachers had more enthusiasm than experience, which gave rise to unsatisfactorily rigid teaching styles. One major, yet familiar, problem was identified by these researchers. This problem is referred to as 'removing the partner'. It reflects the ban on the midwife asking the woman about domestic violence in the presence of her partner or other family members. Suggestions for 'removing' him were ingenious, according to Ward and Spence, but it needed a policy decision to resolve the difficulty. A management directive was implemented requiring that the first five minutes of the 'booking' appointment should be for the woman alone. While a partner might object to this for reasons of being closely involved, his objection might also be due to his abusive behaviour. For this reason community follow-up is essential in such situations.

Conclusion

This chapter has examined the problem of domestic violence, with particular reference to the difficulties with which it is associated during childbearing. This material has shown how it is possible for men to react negatively to their inability to understand and to contribute to the events of childbearing. This negative reaction may manifest itself in some form of violence towards the pregnant or childbearing female partner.

The phenomenon which is domestic violence has been shown to be likely to be facilitated by the increasing involvement of men in childbearing (Garcia and Davidson, 2002). This is due to the abiding presence of the male partner during antenatal care, during labour and, in particular, postnatally, being widely accepted, or even encouraged, by health care providers. The man's close and continuing presence may serve to prevent the woman from seeking help through articulating her abusive situation. He may insist on remaining with her if he suspects that she may disclose his abuse in his absence. In this way the woman does not receive the help to which she is entitled, her difficulty may be aggravated and her situation rendered even more precarious. I venture to suggest that health care providers, by accepting and even encouraging this man's presence, are not only not providing care, but are actually complicit in the abuse of this woman. If this scenario is accurate the reflection on midwifery care is appalling. This is because the midwife, whose job title means 'with woman', is not only not being 'with woman', but may actually be colluding in her abuse.

Chapter 7

Men and loss in childbearing

Introduction

The literature and the childbearing situations which have been examined thus far suggest that there may be some discrepancy, or at least variation, between the rhetoric and the reality of men's contribution to childbearing. The significance of the man's input into one particular aspect of the woman's experience of childbearing is demonstrated by research which has been undertaken in the areas which feature some form of childbearing loss. This research shows the extent to which the man who is the woman's partner may or may not be involved in and affected by the unhappy childbearing event. The research also addresses whether and to what extent he may show any reaction.

In this chapter I consider the impact of loss on the man as a parent, or would-be parent, as well as the impact on him as a health care provider. In order to examine the issues reasonably fully, it is necessary to interpret the term 'loss' quite broadly. Rather than its usually accepted meaning of demise through death, I am using the term to indicate any form of childbearing loss which may provoke a grief reaction. Thus I examine the man's part in the loss of a viable baby, then in the loss of a baby who is miscarried; next is the loss experienced by the man who is in an infertile relationship and, finally, his role in loss through relinquishment for adoption.

Before considering these specific situations of loss, though, it may be helpful to consider some of the theoretical aspects of the man's experience of grief.

Masculine grief

In his important contribution to the literature, Neil Thompson (1997: 76) regrets that what he terms the 'gendered' nature of grief has received so little serious attention. That such attention is necessary became clear to me when a female friend of my mother died after a long illness. My mother was scandalised when the bereaved husband, within hours of the death of his wife, took their dog out for a long walk. This behaviour was both unacceptable and incomprehensible to my mother. She was of the firm opinion that the bereaved person should sit at home, weep and be comforted by visitors. The sad result was that she was doubly disturbed at the time of the death of her friend. This was because her own grief was aggravated by what she considered to be the widower's failure to grieve appropriately. The problem really lay in her perception of his mourning behaviour, which was derived from her own, and her observation of other widows' experience. Thus this example shows that even grief is 'gendered'.

In the absence of authoritative research, Thomson falls back on the use of stereotypes to examine the man's grief and mourning behaviour. The major stereotype features the man's limited ability to articulate his grief in words or emotional behaviour, such as crying. The old admonition 'big boys don't cry' may reflect the tendency of all involved to limit the man's expression of his grief in ways often regarded as stereotypically feminine. These limiting activities may be imposed, not only by those round about, but also by the man himself.

What has become regarded as this typically male pattern of grieving has been shown by Dyregrov (1991) to have become established as early as in boys of school age. Dyregrov found that boys were less able than girls to acknowledge grief and crisis reactions to the sudden death of a teacher. Of particular concern was the inability of boys to express their feelings, even in writing. Their female classmates, on the other hand, were able to write about their reactions as well as the benefits of certain interventions. Dyregrov attributes these differences to the tendency of girls to play more expressively and in pairs, whereas boys involve themselves in competitive, more disciplined group activities. Dyregrov goes on to speculate that the male child learns at an early age to suppress his feelings in the face of danger, whereas the girl learns to confront her complex feelings. He notes that the interventions provided to support bereaved people are designed for women's more open style of grieving. For this reason men are left less well-supported in their grief.

The nature of grief, Thompson (1997) seeks to argue, is an example of a socially constructed aspect of human life. Social constructionism focuses on the interaction of the subjective and the objective interpretations of reality. Thus the importance of fundamental aspects of human life, such as gender, becomes clearly apparent, in the same way that Dyregrov (1991) found that the boy's behaviour both deprived him of the ability to seek emotional support as well as teaching him to reject any support that was offered. Thomson goes on to suggest that the man's more active coping style means that he is likely to receive less help and support. In addition, in the event of the loss of a child, the assumption is likely to be made by those nearby that the bereaved woman is in greater need of support; and this assumption tends to be firmly endorsed by the father's behaviour.

This traditional view of the man's situation has recently been subjected to a certain degree of reinterpretation (Stroebe and Schut, 1995). On the basis of their work with widows, Stroebe and Stroebe (1987) had identified the variation between individuals in the duration and progress of grieving, as well as people's tendency to oscillate and hesitate between stages. This oscillation is seen to demonstrate movement between the more 'feminine' or passive style of grieving, which is combined sequentially with the more active 'masculine' style. Thus these researchers argue that, rather than being purely gender-linked and clearly differentiated, these styles or processes combine in any one individual, irrespective of their gender. This interpretation of coping with grief is now becoming widely known as the 'dual process model'. It features a range of both 'female' loss-oriented activities and a range of 'male' restoration-oriented activities. A combination of these strategies is employed by the grieving person in their attempts to resolve the pain of loss. These two groups of activities are likely to include those listed in Table 7.1.

In this way the gendered nature of grief, which has traditionally been regarded as a dichotomy between the feminine and the masculine, is being reinterpreted more as a dialectic between two distinct coping styles. In understanding a person's grieving, the emphasis is now being related more to the person's position on the trajectory of grief than to their gender.

In the context of this theoretical background, Thompson (1997) argues that oscillation is not only healthy in grieving but also that it is crucial. He goes on to remind the reader that the oscillation should also be balanced between the two types of activity. He maintains that neither the loss-oriented activities nor the restoration-oriented activities *alone* facilitate healthy grief. Thus action to the exclusion of emotion is not healthy. Obviously, the reverse applies equally.

It may be, therefore, that the differentiation between grieving styles is not between different types of people. The distinction may lie within each individual person, regardless of gender, at different times in their experience of grief.

Table 7.1 Dual process activities

Loss-oriented activities	Restoration-oriented activities
• (stereotypically female)	• (stereotypically male)
• grief work	• denial/avoidance
• facing grief	• broken ties/bonds
• breaking bonds/ties	• controlled distraction
• approach	• doing other things
• intrusion	• suppression

The man as a bereaved parent

The role of the bereaved man in situations of loss has all too often been one of 'supporting the womenfolk' (Mander, 1994b). This role, which may have been imposed on the man by society or which may have been self-imposed, has invariably led to him 'being strong' for someone who is widely perceived as being less strong. Research into the male partner's experience of loss in childbearing has tended to support this rather unfortunate and very limited picture of his experience.

The loss of a viable baby

An important example of a study into the father's experience was undertaken in Sweden as part of a large epidemiological survey of care in the event of perinatal loss (Samuelsson *et al.*, 2001). The researchers were able to undertake qualitative interviews with eleven fathers whose babies had died *in utero* between twenty-nine and forty-two weeks of pregnancy. The father's profound sorrow is clearly apparent in this work. Although many of the fathers had some suspicion that the baby's condition was not good, they were still severely distressed when told that the baby was dead. The father's immediate concern, however, was to protect his partner. He believed that he should protect her from the pain of labour and that this would be best achieved by a caesarean operation. The father was accepting, though, when told that this was not necessarily the best solution.

The time lapse between being told of the baby's demise and the onset of labour seems to have been highly valued. Whether this time is best spent in the couple's own home or in the relatively protected environment of the maternity unit remains uncertain. Significantly, these researchers found the father to be disappointed in the information given by staff. This applied, first, on the grounds that he was not included in conversations between the staff and his partner. Second, he felt that the staff tended to resort to technical jargon which he found incomprehensible. For the men, going home without the baby and returning to work were major hurdles.

Samuelsson and colleagues (2001) were able to draw some comparisons between the man's experience of loss and that of the mother. The differences in the couple's experience led to different coping techniques and, hence, to an improvement in their respect for each other. Sometimes, though, different needs and reactions could lead to unfortunate misunderstandings. The relationship appears to have become fraught, as both partners sought to avoid causing further hurt to the other.

These researchers identified the man's wish to locate another man with whom he could share his sorrow. This was especially important in view of men's usual difficulty in 'opening up'. Samuelsson and colleagues recognised the 'special fellowship' (2001: 128) which grew up between the study fathers. Unfortunately, the reader is not given any information about how this fellowship was initiated or how it operated. The men considered that the taking of mementoes, such as photographs, a lock of hair or a footprint, were later found to be 'invaluable' (2001: 128). They considered that these mementoes should always be taken by staff, even when not wanted by the parents. This recommendation is obviously disconcerting, in that it raises a number of ethical issues relating to the parents' autonomy.

The father's traditional perception of his role as being to protect and support his partner emerges yet again from this study. In spite of this, the researchers indicate that the father's major wish is for his needs as a bereaved parent to be recognised by those nearby. While these recommendations are clearly eminently reasonable, they may also appear to be contradictory. It may be that the potentially conflicting nature of the father's aspirations may prove particularly taxing for those staff who provide care. An important finding of this study, though, is the father's preparedness to recognise and to articulate his own needs.

A large longitudinal study was undertaken in Queensland, Australia by Vance and colleagues (2002) to measure 'distress' among couples bereaved by stillbirth, neonatal death or sudden infant death syndrome (SIDS). 'Distress' was measured by quantitative instruments which focused on anxiety, depression and alcohol use. According to Boyle, a large majority of the sample in this study comprised parents bereaved by stillbirth or neonatal death (207 respondents out of 259: 80 per cent) (1997: 62). Yet again, the common problem of accessing and retaining a suitably large sample of men proved challenging. These researchers found that the couple's different expectations of each other's grief were important in the development of their relationship. The father was found to be quite accepting of the woman's severe distress and recognised the significance of her loss. The woman, on the other hand, tended to be unhappy when she perceived the man to be less distressed than she was. In this unfortunate situation, the relationship was found to be likely to begin to deteriorate. This incongruity of the couple's grieving is apparent in the respondents' distress scores. The women's distress declined gradually and consistently over the thirty-month data collection period. This contrasts with the men's, albeit lower scores, which peaked at thirty months.

These two relatively recent studies demonstrate the important issues in research into the man's experience of perinatal death which are still outstanding. The limited recognition of the father's grief and the serious implications of the woman's perception of his grief demonstrate that interventions to help are likely to have long-term benefits.

The loss of a baby who is miscarried

Miscarriage is a topic which serves to throw into sharp relief a number of important issues relating to reproductive loss. This may be because of its relative frequency (Oakley *et al.*, 1990) yet its unexpectedness, as well as its often 'unseen' nature. These factors serve to reduce the significance of miscarriage to many lay people and to many care providers. This, in turn, is likely to aggravate the emotional pain of the couple experiencing it.

The severity of emotional reactions to miscarriage was studied by Beutel and colleagues (1996). This study involved a longitudinal assessment to measure the similarities and differences between the reactions of the woman and of the man. These researchers' four hypotheses focused around men grieving less, expressing their grief less, being less attached to the baby and being instrumental in the woman's psychological recovery. The data generally supported the first three hypotheses. The fourth, however, was less straight-forward. The women in the study reported that they found that the men were initially supportive and reassuring. After about six months, though, the women were found to be dissatisfied with the level of support provided by their partners and that this was associated with an increase in marital conflict. These findings are reminiscent of those of the Queensland study on perinatal loss (Vance et al., 2002), mentioned in the previous section.

An attempt to describe the man's perspective of early miscarriage was also made by Fiona Murphy (1998). She sought to ascertain whether the traditional view of the man endeavouring to be strong for his partner was an accurate reflection of reality in this situation. As with much of the research to which I have referred on men and childbearing, she encountered immense difficulties in locating even a small sample for her phenomenological study. After making two false starts, a 'snowball' technique was eventually used to recruit the five men who acted as her informants. Murphy found that the traditional masculine aspiration of 'being strong' was supported by the data she collected. In addition, there was a tendency among the men to blame the hospital personnel for the unpleasantness of the experience of miscarriage. This blame was applied particularly to the perceived mishandling of the breaking of the bad news of the fetal demise. Murphy was able to describe the coping strategies which the man would seek to employ, such as finding distractions, forgetting, and trying to carry on as normal. This research showed that, to the man, recognising the reality of the baby is crucial to his ability to function sympathetically in the event of miscarriage. The obvious corollary is that this recognition is associated with having 'seen' the baby during an ultrasound scan. In terms of the implications of her findings, Murphy suggests that better follow-up should be provided after a miscarriage. Unfortunately, while regretting nurses' limited input into this man's care, she fails to indicate who would be the best person to provide this follow-up.

Two researchers in England who have also focused on the male partner's experience at the time of miscarriage are Puddifoot and Johnson (1999). These researchers report the findings of the application of the Perinatal Grief Scale (PGS) to a sample of 323 men. This quantitative study involved the collection of data within eight weeks of the miscarriage event. These researchers report the widespread assumption that the father is impervious to the pain of loss. Their data, however, contradict this assumption by finding that the grief levels measured in the men were similar to those of the women. This study went on to show that there is a strong and positive correlation between the depth of the man's grief and both the duration of the pregnancy and having seen the ultrasound scan. This latter point resonates with Fiona Murphy's findings in the context of early miscarriage (see above).

Following the findings of the PGS, Puddifoot and Johnson discuss their observation that involvement in this research project may have served as a cathartic experience for the man who was grieving. This observation is interesting, especially in view of the obvious enthusiasm of the men to be involved in this study. Whereas Fiona Murphy (1998; see above) recounted her serious difficulty in recruiting even five men respondents, and research mentioned throughout this book has endorsed that difficulty, John Puddifoot and Martin Johnson were able to recruit 323 men. These researchers regret that the response rate to the distribution of their research packs was only 56 per cent. The reader is only able to surmise why these researchers were successful in their recruitment, where others failed so abysmally.

In another publication by Puddifoot and Johnson (1997), they report the qualitative findings of their study in the North of England. By way of endorsement of my last observation, these researchers report having been in a position to randomly select twenty men from among forty-two volunteers to be interviewed. These researchers were told of a culture of non-communication of the man with his male peers. This inability to share his experiences applied even to the men who had gone through a similar loss as recently as two weeks previously.

The men found that they were being forced to subscribe to a culture in which they are regarded as strong, and showing their feelings of sorrow is not permitted. The expression of grief is widely viewed as a self-indulgence. Interestingly, it is not only men who enforced acquiescence to this cultural norm. One grieving father told of being reprimanded by his own mother; when on finding him tearful, she said: 'that I was being selfish and had to pull myself together before I upset [my partner]' (1997: 839).

In terms of the man's communication with his partner, views varied between two extremes. On the one hand the man was silent through his fear of saying the wrong thing and causing further upset. On the other hand the man was silent because he considered that the couple's shared feelings were sufficiently eloquent, that their feelings were beyond words and that there was no need to resort to speech. Uncertainty remains, though, of whether the woman partner would be in a suitable frame of mind to be able to distinguish between these two extremes.

Serious questions were raised by Puddifoot and Johnson about the legitimacy or illegitimacy of the man's feelings of sorrow. The researchers suggest that, due to their perception that the demonstration of grief is not appropriate for a man in the event of a miscarriage, these men were effectively in denial of their feelings. They resorted to justification of their lack of grief by regarding the miscarried baby as having been something other than a 'real baby' or a 'proper baby' (1997: 840). An element of blame was bound up with these forms of justification, in which the woman was perceived as over-reacting to the miscarriage:

'She just likes making a fuss.'

'She talks about it as if we had actually lost a baby, but we haven't because it had never been born alive.'

The justification of the loss through miscarriage tended towards the traditional forms of rationalisation to the effect that it was 'Nature's way' [of disposing of a less than perfect baby] (1997: 842). This element of blame was even more overt for some of the men. One man, jealous of his wife's premarital sexual experience, suggested that these activities were responsible for the miscarriage. Another blamed her active social life:

'She did keep going to the club and who knows what they do on their Friday nights out?'
'Well her smoking won't have helped, would it?'
'Look we do our bit right, then it's up to them, isn't it?'

(1997: 842)

The men also reported some degree of self-blame. This sometimes took the form of an inability to correct a situation that was going seriously wrong, which was perceived as a serious threat: I stood like a lemming not knowing what to do . . . just like a little boy who can't find his mummy' (1997: 841). Such feelings of regression were clearly a threat to the man's self-esteem, as was the risk that he might lose the woman's high regard: 'I'm sure that I will have lost some respect in her eyes now, and rightly so' (ibid.).

For some of the men the feelings aroused by the miscarriage were even more profound. Questions emerged about the meaning or pointlessness of life and the fundamental threat exerted by a loss such as this. Puddifoot and Johnson summarise their findings in terms of the men's 'unfinished business' which is left over from their own and their partners' past experiences. Some of these relate to childhood, whereas other left-over experiences are more recent. These researchers regret the man's inability to find a role in the event of a miscarriage, which is generally defined as a 'female event'. Puddifoot and Johnson conclude that the man is effectively in what they term a 'double bind'. This amounts to the man feeling that anything he does will inevitably aggravate the unhappy situation, so his solution is to do nothing. Unfortunately, this has the effect of aggravating the situation, because it causes him to appear to be uncaring. The researchers' analysis, however, fails to take account of the effect of the time warp in which women have become able to talk more openly about unhappy events. Men, however, have either excluded themselves or have been excluded from these conversations.

According to Puddifoot and Johnson, some men suffer from serious emotional pain as a consequence.

The loss experienced by the man in an infertile relationship

The man in an involuntarily infertile relationship has invariably received less attention than his female partner (Glover *et al.*, 1998). This may be because of the traditional assumption that the woman, formerly sometimes labelled as being 'barren', has been considered to be the 'guilty' party in these circumstances.

The lack of research attention to the role of the man in an infertile relationship in which the woman is being treated may be an example of this bias. An attempt was made by Harris (1994) to redress this imbalance through a research study. She found that the level of the man's instrumental support and the level of his emotional support interacted to create a range of possible responses to the couple's infertility:

- The man offering a high level of both instrumental and emotional support was termed an 'activist', as he was both sympathetic and effective.
- The man offering neither form of support was termed an 'aggravator'. This was because he appeared to exacerbate the couple's increasingly negative perception of the infertility problem.
- The 'co-operator' was found to offer practical support, but not sympathy.
- The man termed the 'sideliner' scored high on emotional support, but was devoid of any real agency.

Thus Glover and colleagues' criticism (1998) of the dearth of research and other attention to the man's experience of infertility is gradually beginning to be addressed. This process is more advanced in other cultures, where the stigma of male infertility may be even more distressing than in the West (Lee and Chu, 2001; Lee *et al.*, 2001). The work of Greil (1997), however, attempted to critically analyse the existing literature. He found that the woman is more likely to be seriously affected by the couple's infertility than the man. This applies in a number of ways, such as lower self-esteem, more depression, lower life satisfaction and more self-blame (1997: 1694). In making comparisons between the man's and the woman's experience of infertility, it is usually assumed that couples attending for infertility treatment constitute a suitably balanced sample. This form of sampling may be problematic, as Greil observes that the partners of men who decline to participate tend to be much more distressed than their peers. Thus, a form of sampling bias may be inherent. Such methodological problems are also found in this man's greater tendency to lie, his self-aggrandisement and his denial of psychological distress. These problems are inevitably magnified further by the under-representation of non-whites and lower socio-economic groups in these samples.

It is widely accepted that the infertile couple may need to grieve the loss of their *potential* child (Mander, 1994: 53). This view has long been acknow-ledged, since it originated with the pioneering work of Frank (1984) and Menning (1982). This egalitarian view, however, has been challenged more recently. Glover and colleagues (1998) concede that the woman who is infertile tends to respond to her situation as if to a bereavement, by demonstrating high levels of depression. The man in an infertile relationship, however, reacts to the situation somewhat differently. For the man, depression is the less likely reaction. His response is more likely to involve anxiety than depression. In their 1996 publication Glover and colleagues report their study using the Hospital Anxiety and Depression Scale (HADS). They found that the infertile man's anxiety was measured at approximately five times the level expected in the general population. These researchers' longitudinal study showed that, with time, the man became more and more convinced that his partner was to blame for their infertility. At the same time, the man became increasingly likely to assume that a pregnancy would resolve the wide range of problems which the couple was experiencing.

Glover and colleagues (1998) argue, on the basis of these findings, that the man's anxiety response suggests that he perceives the infertility within his relationship more as a threat than as a loss. For this reason, these researchers suggest that a pregnancy is only likely to resolve the problems found in this man's partner. Their subsequent data (Glover *et al.*, 1999) show that the pregnancy (which occurred in 30 per cent of the couples in the sample) did not significantly affect the man's anxiety. Thus pregnancy may not be the answer to this man's anxiety, his self-blame and his uncertainties about his manliness. These authors suggest that this man's problems may be much more deep-seated and less easily amenable to resolution.

The man and loss through relinquishment for adoption

The role of the 'menfolk' in the childbearing process was thrown into sharp relief by a study of the midwife's care of the mother who relinquishes her baby for adoption (Mander, 1995). As well as interviews with experienced midwives, a series of in-depth interviews was undertaken with twenty-three women who were either relinquishing or had relinquished a baby for adoption. Because part of the research method involved asking the woman to tell her 'story', background information about her circumstances was provided which informed her total experience of her relinquishment. The two men, who were almost invariably mentioned by the woman, were the father of the baby and the woman's own father. In spite of immense variability in the women's experiences, certain crucial themes emerged which related to these two groups of men.

The father of the baby

The role of the baby's father fell quite consistently into one of two very different groups. Some of the women regarded the role and the relationship with the baby's father as crucially important to her and her well-being. These important relationships tended to be temporarily interrupted by the pregnancy, the birth and the relinquishment. The alternative scenario was that, for practical purposes, this man's role and hence any relationship was, or quickly became, non-existent. The former father was, although not part of the family in the traditional formal sense, part of the woman's family in everything but name. For a larger proportion of the mothers, however, the father of the relinquished baby was of virtually negligible significance in her experience. This applied to such an extent that he may not even have been mentioned in the woman's account of her experience.

For a very small number of the women, these insignificant men tended to be part of a relationship that was brief, exclusively sexual and has been referred to as a 'back of the chip shop job'. This was demonstrated in Barbara's account (all names are fictitious). The women's names were changed to maintain their anonymity and the menfolk were all given the same names for the same reason and to avoid distraction.

> BARBARA: I didn't know what was going on. OK I wasn't *that* stupid, but at the same time you don't. I don't know where he lived. He lived outside [the city], but certainly in some village.

While such a brief encounter may verge on being a stereotype, for a larger proportion of the women the pregnancy resulted from a long-term relationship. Such established relationships were seriously damaged to the extent of being ended as a result of the conception and pregnancy. The conception and relinquishment engendered differing and unequal levels of antagonism between the woman and the baby's father. The women's accounts suggest that there was considerable variation in their perceptions of the extent to which the mother or the father rejected the other.

> WILMA: He was not a nice person and the conception occurred after what you might call a seduction, but was more like a rape . . . I had known him for seven years. He was known as a rotter, but I was very much in love with him.

> GINA: I had no more contact with the father of the child. But I never told him either, so it is something that I have kept under the surface all these years.

> JESSICA: I wasn't taking any precautions and neither was he. [Sexual intercourse] was a one off and unfortunately I was caught out. He

disowned me, he refused to admit that he was the father of the child, which I found hurt me a lot, although we were not in love and we were certainly not planning to get married.

QUELIA: The baby's father and I knew each other for a very long time. He was still around and he pleaded with me for the first five months of my pregnancy for us to get married. I just wasn't interested. It was when I was pregnant that I realised that I didn't love him as much as I thought I did.

For some of the women, though, the conception and relinquishment did not diminish her growing affection for the father of her baby. This effect operated in spite, or possibly because of, her parent's disapproval and their attempts to control and terminate their daughter's relationship with him:

NADIA: I became pregnant when I was at college. I met the one who's now my husband when I was 17. He became my stable boy friend. I became pregnant when I was just eighteen. Billy was forbidden to see me, but while I was [away] I wrote to him every day. I actually got engaged to Billy in the August and it was in October I signed the [adoption] papers and I married Billy a year later.

HILDA: Billy still today swears he did not know anything about the bairn. He had not been told about him . . . My Mum and Dad did not want him to have anything to do with me they just wanted him to leave me and let me hae the bairn and sort o' get on wi' it. Eventually me and Billy got married.

Thus for a small number of the women the conception comprised one episode in a long-lasting, albeit turbulent, yet for some, still ongoing relationship:

ROSA: I had been going out with the baby's father for quite a while. It was all rather stupid, because I married the baby's father afterwards anyway.

VERA: When I found out that I was pregnant I felt that I had to part from the father of my baby. Some time later, after I gave my baby away, I met [the baby's] father again and we were still in love. He was angry with me for giving his baby away but I had had no choice. The baby had been conceived in love and we still loved each other. He asked me to marry him.

It is apparent that the role of the father of the baby varied between the interrupted ongoing relationship and the terminated or non-existent relationship.

The findings of this study correspond closely with those of Marck (1994) in her research into women experiencing unexpected pregnancy. In both of these studies the baby's father's role may be appropriately summarised, in Marck's words, as being 'extraneous'.

The mother's father

Compared with the baby's father, a generally far more significant contributor to the relinquishing mother's experience was her father; that is, the grandfather of the baby who was relinquished. The mother's relationship with her father was typically that he loved and admired her (Bronfenbrenner, 1961), to the extent that her father tended to idealise his daughter or to put her on a 'pedestal':

> TANYA: He called me 'Princess' all his life and I was his little princess.

REACTION TO THE NEWS OF THE PREGNANCY

It is hardly surprising in view of the father's doting on his daughter that the news of the conception shocked him beyond anything the woman could possibly have expected. The father's expression of his shock took differing forms:

> QUELIA: My Dad, I think he was stunned into silence with the shock – his daughter could actually let this happen to her, he's kind of had me up on a pedestal to this day, but that time I kind of knocked myself off it.

> TANYA: I'm surprised you didn't hear him in Edinburgh. He went berserk. He came through [to my room] and he started calling me all these really horrible names, I remember he called me a slut . . . it was just the way he said it. He was absolutely horrified, absolutely disgusted with me, y'know, for being in that condition. It was terrible, y'know, he was not going to let up, he was going on and on and on. 'Cos my mother was in tears and it was she who eventually said 'That is it, enough'.

With time for quiet reflection each woman was able to come to understand the rationale for her father's powerful and acutely painful negative reaction to the news of her pregnancy. For some fathers, the women thought that the realisation of their daughter's maturity and forthcoming independence had been impressed on him in an unexpectedly blatant and abrupt way. This realisation, they understood, continued to be a long-term source of misgiving:

> QUELIA: I think he realised that he'd lost his wee girl. She's now a woman, she's pregnant herself and all of a sudden this wee girl is not

a wee girl any more – she's a young woman now, with responsibilities of her own. We never actually discussed it properly, my Dad and I.

For other fathers, their difficulty lay in the stark and bewildering contrast between their previous idealisation of the daughter and the new reality. This contrast may be described in terms of a 'depedestalisation':

> TANYA: [he reacted so badly] probably because [he couldn't understand] how could I have done that, let him down like that. I think he felt so badly let down by me.

PREGNANCY DECISION-MAKING

The father's adverse reaction to his daughter's pregnancy is reflected in the instrumental role which he sought to play in decision-making concerning the future of the pregnancy and of the child. This search for an instrumental role may constitute a form of compensation for the man's inability to prevent her pregnancy. The initial decision concerning the continuation of the pregnancy comprised a knee-jerk reaction by some of the fathers that a termination of pregnancy was the only realistic solution. For a variety of reasons the woman often did not recognise the pregnancy until it was well advanced. This meant that termination was not a possibility, even for those mothers who conceived after the enactment of the 1967 UK legislation:

> FRANCESCA: The scan confirmed that I was 6 months pregnant so I knew I would have to go through with it. Dad was ill with worry. I was away with it. We spoke to an obstetrician and Dad asked for me to have an abortion. The obstetrician refused. Dad said he would get it done privately, and the obstetrician said that that was impossible 'cos it was illegal.

> TANYA: My father had obviously . . . phoned his sister. They were very close – my father and his sister. I think it was her doctor we went to see actually. I think she must've phoned her doctor – it was a lady doctor and we went along and she confirmed the pregnancy. And I can remember [my father] asking her if there wasn't any way I could have an abortion? . . . And she said 'no' because there wasn't really any reason for it. . . . So it was decided that I would just have to carry on with the pregnancy and have the baby adopted. This was all decided for me, by the way, nobody asked me.

The decision-making role of the father became a reality when, after the possibility of a termination of pregnancy had been excluded, the mother was presented, like Tanya (above), with adoption as the only feasible solution:

DEBRA: It was not my decision – it was suggested, it was always suggested. It probably started with my father.

FRANCESCA: When Dad found out I couldn't have an abortion, he said 'Adoption, adoption' and I said 'Yes, yes'. Me being so small and young, I went along with the plans for the baby to be adopted in order to avoid further hassle to my father.

CLARA: I was forced into [adoption] by my father.

THE GRANDFATHER AND THE BABY

After the birth of the baby, the new grandfather's behaviour tended to continue in the same pattern established during pregnancy:

DEBRA: My Father was uncomfortable looking at the baby. He came with my Mother to visit but he wouldn't look at her or hold her.

SANDRA: [My Mother is interested in the newborn baby] but my father just says 'How are things going?' 'Are they finalised?' He just wants to see the adoption finalised.

For some of the mothers, though, her father's consistency was more positive, helpful and appreciated:

KARA: I went home (after the birth and relinquishment) and my Mother and everybody was really fine. . . . My Dad came in from work and he gave me a big hug.

RM: Does he do that often?

KARA: Seldom. This was unusual. Because he was really upset about me. I knew because for the whole of the time that I was pregnant he hardly spoke.

LENA: I love my Dad. He made me feel as if it wasn't the end of the world, 'cos my Mom always made me feel I was the only one in the world that had had a kid at fourteen.

LONG-TERM EFFECTS

In the same way as signs of emotion were generally suppressed by most of the fathers, verbal communication relating to the baby tends to continue to be restricted. This may be more a reflection of the openness of functioning of the family system, rather than a personality characteristic of the father:

> QUELIA: I've never really discussed her. My father is about the only one that ever really talks about her at any time. My Dad says she's still his grandchild. It was coming up to her first birthday before my Dad and me got round to talking about her in the house, my Dad was wondering how I was feeling and I was wondering how he was feeling.

When such a closed pattern of communication becomes established within the family, the family members face great difficulty in overcoming it. Nadia was concerned that this form of 'unfinished business' should be dealt with while there was still an opportunity; that is, while her father was still alive:

> NADIA: He has *never* spoken to me about [my relinquishment]. The whole episode was *never ever* mentioned. *Never.* The fact that the fostering fees had been returned was the only mention ever made of it by my father. About twelve years ago I raised it with him and he seemed quite relieved at that. I think my Dad is still upset about it though.

In the same way as the father's helpful and supportive behaviour, as well as any non-communicative behaviour, tended to continue beyond the birth and relinquishment, his desire to help by protecting his daughter persisted. This was usually viewed by the daughter as misplaced and unhelpful protection, which served mainly to prevent her from continuing her life as she wished, by building the relationships she preferred and maintaining her options for contact:

> FRANCESCA: My father warned the others in the family not to help me to keep the baby by giving me somewhere to live. He wanted to prevent me from 'ruining my life any more'.

> TANYA: I told my first husband, it was just after he had proposed to me. When we told Dad that we wanted to get married he said that he was surprised that anyone would want to marry me after they knew I had had a baby adopted. I can't help wondering if there was a feeling at the back of my mind that I'd better marry him in case it was my last chance.

> BARBARA: You have to register a birth within so many days . . . I registered her Andrea. . . . the Registrar said 'What's the surname?' And I can remember to this day just going to say Jones-Donald. My Dad said 'No, it's Donald'. I know, and I knew then, that he was doing that to protect me in future. But sometimes it bugs me because, I think,

you are making the path – if she wants to come and find me – you are making the path a bit harder. I think that is what he was thinking of at the time.

The father's initial reaction to the news of his daughter's pregnancy was invariably negative, but to differing degrees. The duration of his negative response was variable. The reasons for this powerfully negative response may be attributed to a variety of factors. The first, mentioned by Martin (1987), relates to the father's need to be a successful parent. In the success-oriented world of men, a daughter's apparently unwanted pregnancy may constitute the ultimate evidence of his failure as a male parent. The second reason is associated with the father's increasingly obvious failure to control his daughter's behaviour. Martin considers that the father's fears focus most strongly on those activities in which errors are least easily solved. For Martin the examples include sex, drugs and alcohol. The father's inability to control his daughter's sexual behaviour, perhaps indicating slipping control in other areas of his life, may be partly responsible for the overwhelmingly adverse reaction which the mothers in this sample encountered.

From this work, it is clear that her own father features prominently in the mother's experience of relinquishment. Occasionally he was able to provide much-needed and appreciated support, but more often he assumed a decision-seeking, decision-taking and decision-imposing role. This reflected the ongoing relationships within the family, had serious implications for the future of those relationships and affected the mother's potential for relationships with any future partners as well as her child.

For this vulnerable childbearing woman, though, the input of the menfolk close to her was not helpful to her. The behaviour of both groups of men, at least of those who remained in contact, varied between the absent, the relatively neutral and the totally negative. This research shows that, unlike the woman's mother and the woman's friends, the welfare of this vulnerable childbearing woman was not the main concern of these menfolk.

The man as a care provider

The man who provides care in situations of loss has attracted less attention, and particularly less research attention, than have partners and fathers in situations of childbearing loss.

In the late twentieth century, interest in the experience of childbearing loss developed rapidly. This interest was fuelled by a serendipitous finding by Bourne (1968). In a study of the causes of perinatal death, this researcher found that the general practitioners who were contacted were quite unable to recall any cases of perinatal death in their practices. On the basis of this observation, Bourne concluded that the general practitioner's reaction to such a death was so adverse that he was not able to cope with it. For this reason the general practitioner would effectively obliterate it from his consciousness, from his mind and from his memory.

The work of Moulder, thirty years later, demonstrates the extent to which medical men have been able to learn from the ample research and other literature which had been produced in the interim:

> I'm not sure it has a huge impact emotionally because I manage to distance myself. That's how I deal with things.

> You can be really understanding and sympathetic and not yet feel emotional about it yourself.

> I suppose I detach myself from it quite a lot really. I don't really dwell on it . . . there's no point.

(Moulder, 1998: 186)

This strategy, referred to as 'distancing' by Moulder's first informant, features regularly in the disaster research literature (Ursano *et al.*, 1995). It is recognised as a coping strategy, which involves the precise demarcation and separation of personal from professional events. This strategy operates for groups, for example, military body handlers, who socialise with their peers and are unable, due to the nature of their work, to share their work anxieties with their partners. In my recent study of the midwife's care of the mother who dies (Mander, 2001b) one of my informants (Midwife 17) reported that her daughter, a paramedic, had advised her to make use of this strategy:

> She says when we are faced with that sort of thing, because we are nurses as well, we put our nursing mode on. That's a coping strategy in itself, she says. You sort of withdraw yourself from the emotion and you sort of go into professional mode and you help pass the instruments and so on and so forth.

This strategy may also be termed 'compartmentalisation'. The research in which it has been identified was undertaken on samples of male personnel involved in disaster events. It incorporates certain stereotypically male characteristics, such as the more 'masculine' forms of coping and peer support (Etzion, 1984).

Even Midwife 17, though, soon realised that this strategy is far from realistic for the midwife: 'And [the midwives are] devastated and all these things, but they don't have a professional compartment to put it into 'cos they haven't developed one.' This midwife concluded that it is the lack of experience of traumatic work-related events which prevents the midwife's use of this coping strategy. There is an alternative explanation, though. It may be that this strategy is quite alien to female coping. This is because, as Etzion has observed, women are less likely to seek and find routine support among their work colleagues. She maintains that women's support lies in their "traditional" or "real" role as wives and mothers' (1984). Thus the 'oneness' of the woman's life becomes apparent and any possibility of compartmentalisation is impeded.

Thus it is necessary for me to suggest that the coping strategies which appear to be employed successfully by emergency personnel in disaster situations may also be appropriate for use in situations of loss in health care.

Conclusion

In this chapter the research literature has been used to examine the man's experience of loss in childbearing. As interest in this topic is not yet well-developed, the research literature-base is still similarly small. In spite of this, the picture which emerges is fairly consistent across the areas of loss which have to date been subjected to research scrutiny. At the risk of being accused of stereotyping, the picture is one of the man having his own agenda. Further, it seems that this agenda is not necessarily the same as that of the woman partner who may be sharing the loss or the female personnel who are caring for her.

Chapter 8

How to help – the midwife's role

In this chapter I focus, once again, on both the man as a father as well as on the man as a care provider. The situation of these men during the child-bearing process has been critically examined in the preceding chapters. I now refocus our attention to build on the earlier chapters, with a view to making recommendations to remedy any unsatisfactory aspects of the situation in which the man finds himself. In order to do this, I will attempt to analyse the proposals which have been advanced in order to assess their feasibility and effectiveness. The proposals have related mainly to the needs of the man becoming a father as opposed to the man as a care provider. The proposals have sought to address aspects such as his education and support. These aspects, though, have been addressed from various angles, including from policy, practice and personal viewpoints.

Throughout this chapter, I focus as far as is possible on the research evidence. On occasions the research evidence is lacking, unclear or otherwise deficient; only then do I fall back on the more plentiful supply of anecdotes, personal experiences and opinions.

Helping the father

In this section the focus is on the sources of assistance available to the new father. These sources may be tapped during pregnancy, at childbirth, and in the early days, weeks, months and years of being a father.

Supporting the father

The research literature on the support available to the father is limited. This may be due to the widespread assumption that he does not need support because his role is merely to be there to provide support for his partner. Whether and to what extent this assumption is valid remains to be seen. This assumption, and the associated lack of literature, may be derived in part from the North American situation, where much of the basic supportive care for the woman in labour is provided by her partner. In spite, or perhaps because of, this, the randomised controlled trials on support in childbearing have paid scant attention to the father. These researchers have preferred to focus their attention on a range of exclusively female carers. The most notable, or notorious, of these carers is the 'doula' (Mander, 2001b).

There are a small number of important exceptions to this observation of the lack of literature on support of the father. The first assumes a midwife-oriented stance to consider both practice- and policy-related issues (Lester and Moorsom, 1997). These authors advocate that the midwife should be in a position to provide informational and emotional support for the father. They then go on to recommend certain policy changes. These include the establishment of men-only support groups, as well as childbirth education sessions and antenatal clinics which are workplace based and held during evenings and at weekends. Lester and Moorsom continue by recommending a further, more contentious, policy change, which permits the father to 'room in' while the mother and baby are in hospital. This latter recommendation may initially appear to be seriously contentious. It soon becomes apparent, however, that it will rapidly become less controversial as the duration of hospital stay grows even shorter.

The second exception is found in the work of Tom Beardshaw (2001). After contributing to a book on single parenthood, Beardshaw became Campaigns Manager of the charity Fathers Direct. Whether the *double entendre* in the name of this charity is deliberate is not known. In this role he has written about the support which the midwife may provide for the father around the time of the birth of the child. He describes the father's three key roles in terms of, first, providing support in both emotional and practical ways for the new mother. He claims that the partner is the woman's 'main source' of emotional support. The father's second role is to provide practical help with child care. Drawing on the 1978 work of Frodi and colleagues, he asserts that this role is facilitated by the slightly ambiguous fact that fathers are 'naturally as good with babies as women' (2001: 478). The third and probably least contentious role is the father as breadwinner, which is explained as the reason for his prolonged absence from the family home.

Beardshaw goes on to confess that the father may constitute a 'burden' to overstretched health professionals. This issue is not addressed in his paradoxical argument which both praises the benefits of paternal involvement and asserts the need for appropriate preparation for this role. This preparation, however, requires that certain needs should be addressed. The needs he catalogues, though, must be recognised as not being no-cost, or even low-cost, activities:

- Information
- Involvement in discussions
- Preparation class
- Support for practical involvement in labour

- Allowing father into hospital to provide support
- Ensuring father is present when skills and/or information are transmitted
- A national strategy for information relating to paternity leave.

Thus, crucial to Beardshaw's argument is that the role of the father is best supported by meeting the information needs of men through specifically focused materials and activities.

This demand for information for the father is reminiscent of one of the major research-based findings of Singh and Newburn (2000). These researchers sought to identify the support and information needs of men becoming fathers. They accessed a sample of men through the use of the database created by 'Bounty', which is a sampling organisation. This database provided the details of the childbearing woman, to whom the self-completion postal question-naire was sent, together with a request to pass the material on to her partner. The pregnancy questionnaire elicited a response rate of a mere 37 per cent, although only 35.5 per cent of the responses were suitable for analysis. The postnatal questionnaire produced 463 responses, which is just 20 per cent of the original population. The researchers contend that these response rates are not as unrepresentative as they may appear at first sight. This is due to the fact that some of the women recipients of the questionnaires would have been without partners. A further problem with this sample is the strange distribution of the responses, which shows a bimodal distribution, peaking in socio-economic classes II and IV.

The men who were included in this slightly unusual sample, however, articulated clearly their need for information on:

- *In pregnancy*
  - Maternity service choices
  - Mood swings in pregnancy

- *In labour*
  - What to expect/interventions
  - How to help their partner
  - Pain control
  - Movement

- *After the birth*
  - Postnatal depression
  - Money/benefits
  - Sex

- *About the baby*
  - Coping with crying
  - Coping with baby and other children
  - Crying and sleeping

- Bathing
- Effects on relationship
- Starting solids
- Mixed feeding
- Assisting breast-feeding
- Amounts of formula.

While some of these information needs, such as postnatal sex and the baby's effects on the relationship, may be more obscure, many of these topics would be easily found in published material, including being on the Internet.

Educating the father

It may be that Beardshaw's plea for more, and more appropriate, informational support to be provided for the father is in reality an appeal for the revision of childbirth education. Such a plea seems to be to make the content more relevant to him. It may equally be to include him more specifically, or to make the general ambience of childbirth education more father-friendly.

In order to benefit the childbirth education provided by Swedish midwives, Hallgren and her colleagues undertook a phenomenological study involving eleven fathers (1999; see Chapter 4, pp. 84–5, this volume). The success of the childbirth education in facilitating the couple's close relationship is reflected in the major concept which emerged from this study. This concept was 'vital involvement', which relates to the couple's psychosocial development and which manifested itself in their shared feelings of 'we' contributing to the birth. Childbirth education was found to be effective in preparing the father to take an active role at the birth.

Hallgren and colleagues found that a perhaps unwelcome benefit of childbirth education was that the father was able to cope more easily with his own powerlessness and the meaninglessness of some events during the birth. A disadvantage of the woman-centred childbirth education which the midwives espoused was that a rift was caused between the partners after their earlier mutually supportive educational activity. This form of education also led to exaggerated and unrealistic expectations of the protective role which the father would be able to offer during childbirth. Problems were identified, too, of conflicting information and a lack of guidance or support. Perhaps more surprisingly, anxiety arose due to the man being left alone with his partner in labour. The fathers interviewed gave a strong impression of having felt unprepared for their role at the birth. This manifested itself in the men experiencing difficulty in coping with the intensity and the unpredictability of the process of childbirth. These difficulties applied particularly to the length of time involved and the woman's labour pain. Acute difficulties arose due to the woman's actions during her labour and the man's reactions to them.

The childbirth educators had anticipated that the man would be prepared to assume an ideal role which would be mutually supportive. This ideal role was found to be too difficult for the men. Instead, each man resorted to the more traditional, passive role of being a witness to the birth. As a result of this passive role he allowed the midwife to provide the support which he had planned to offer to the woman. On the basis of these findings, Hallgren and her colleagues recommend that the midwife should monitor the man's 'vital involvement' during both the pregnancy and childbirth. They suggest that the midwife should be prepared to intervene to prevent any untoward side effects.

While this Swedish study endeavoured to improve the father's experience through more appropriate childbirth education, it is clear that not all of the researchers' aims were accomplished. Obviously, the father's 'vital involvement' was a benefit, but this did not overcome the systematic problems encountered by the father during the labour and birth.

Other unexpected effects of childbirth education were identified by the fathers involved in a research project in England (Greenhalgh et al., 2000). These researchers found that they were able to categorise the fathers into two groups depending on their styles of coping with stressful situations, the obvious example being their partner's labour. The first major group was referred to as the 'Monitors', as these men sought to keep a close watch on the progress of labour by seeking copious information. The other group of men were labelled the 'Blunters', due to their anxiety tending to cause them to distract attention away from the crucial activities of the birth. The data analysis showed that the Blunters who had previously attended childbirth education tended to be the group who were the more dissatisfied with the birth experience. Greenhalgh and her colleagues focus on the man's anxiety and the way this may be affected by childbirth education. This highly respected group of researchers argue that, rather than being universally beneficial, it may be that childbirth education actually serves to aggravate the anxiety experienced by many fathers (2000: 183).

The impression which emerges from the important research projects examined so far is that childbirth education may not be helpful to some fathers. In fact, it is possible that it may even be counter-productive.

'Fathers-only' childbirth education

As well as these general attempts to improve the father's experience though better childbirth education, more specific tactics have been employed. One of these tactics, which is suggested not infrequently, is 'fathers-only' classes. The attraction of such a system would lie in the focus being indisputably on the father, rather than his being regarded merely as some kind of appendage. On the basis of her wealth of experience of teaching childbirth education, Andrea Robertson (1999) outlines some techniques to involve men more effectively. As well as practical problem-solving exercises, she outlines some questionably realistic activities which are intended to lead to him being confident when in the labour ward. More likely to be effective, though, are the men-only group discussions which provide the men with a safe environment in which to explore their own emotional needs.

Following her research (see Chapter 3, p. 74, this volume), Nina Smith (1999a, 1999b) dismisses the possibility of fathers-only classes as being unacceptable. It is necessary to question whether this outright dismissal is because such classes might force men to address, or even confront, their own deep inner feelings, rather than just acting in the usual rather peripheral supportive role.

The concept of a fathers-only childbirth education class formed the basis of a quasi-experimental study by Diemer (1997). This study involved a comparison between traditional childbirth classes, with their focus on the mother, with the innovative father-focused classes. The principle of single-sex group work underpinned these sessions, together with positive attempts to involve the fathers in group discussion. The fathers were taught strategies which would help them to locate and recruit support for themselves and to increase their own social networks. Diemer indicates that there were abundant opportunities for the fathers to 'open up' about their feelings and their experiences. In spite of this, the curriculum continued to present a substantial proportion of traditional material on the father's support for his partner.

Following her analysis of her data, Diemer found that the changes in the behaviour of the men who attended the 'father-focused' classes were 'not as extensive as expected' (1997: 290). The data, however, did show increases in the couple's mutual understanding, in the man's participation in house-work, in his coping through the use of social support, and in his obtaining information from his partner's physician. Clearly these results represent some movement in the direction of meeting the father's needs through childbirth education. The fact that the findings did not reach the desired levels of significance is disappointing.

Men's criticisms of childbirth education

If childbirth education is ever to meet the needs of the father, it is crucial that attention should be paid to, and action taken on, the comments of the men who have attended. All too often evaluations and feedback are merely a 'letting off steam' exercise rather than part of a quality assurance cycle to ensure a high standard of learning experience. A number of research projects, while not necessarily focusing solely on fathers' feedback, have included reference to them; this feedback may be valuable in assessing whether and how men's experience of childbearing may be ameliorated.

A Finnish study indicates the large proportion of parents in that country who attend for childbirth education, although it is referred to as 'family training'. Effectively, attenders comprise all pregnant women and 75 per cent of their partners (Vehvilainen-Julkunen, 1995: 731). This researcher outlines previous criticisms of the father's experience of childbirth education. The major criticism, as implied by the study in England by Singh and Newburn (2000), has related to information, or rather the lack of it. Fathers in previous studies were critical that they had not been given information about life with a new baby. Similarly, they felt that material on the interaction between the parents and between the parent and the child had been lacking (Vehvilainen-Julkunen, 1995: 732). The fathers in the earlier studies had sought more teaching on the care of the newborn baby. Fathers have been generally critical of the information on the grounds that it had been contradictory and out of date. Further, attention to psychological issues has also been criticised for being inadequate.

Following her analysis of the literature, the research by Vehvilainen-Julkunen (1995) involved the distribution of a questionnaire to 189 mothers and 127 fathers, by nurses handing them out when the baby was 9 weeks old. This study found that there were no major differences between the views of the mothers and the fathers about childbirth education. All the respondents attached more importance to postnatal events and found that antenatal topics, such as an abnormal course of pregnancy and the advance hospital visit, were less significant. The mother–father relationship was also judged to be less important. It is necessary to question whether these findings relate to the timing of the questionnaire, in that the parents of a 9-week-old baby may have preoccupations other than events during pregnancy.

In her grounded theory study of the part played by childbirth education in men's transition to fatherhood, Smith (1999a) found a more complex picture of experiences and needs. She undertook semi-structured interviews with eighteen fathers whose children were aged between 4 weeks and 13 weeks. Smith initially sought a sample incorporating 'a wide social cross section' (1999a: 23). She blames the homogeneity of her sample, though, on the fact that she did not have funds to travel outside London and, hence, the men were all 'professional and well-educated'. This is exemplified by the fact that fourteen of the men (78 per cent) were graduates (Smith, 1999b: 328).

Following data analysis (1999b: 329), Smith found that what emerged as important to her informants was 'the whole birth thing'. They did not seek mere 'medical facts and technical knowledge' (1999a: 24). The transmission of such basic information led to severe disillusionment among some informants on the grounds of its superficiality. Smith explains that her respondents were seeking to understand a holistic picture of the nature of birth. What they seem to have been presented with was criticised in terms of its focus on 'biological processes and medical procedures'.

The emotional content of her interviews with these men is implicit in Smith's account of her study. She states: 'the need to debrief about their birth experiences was very evident' (1999a: 24). Whether this 'need to debrief' related to disappointment, or anger, or a combination of the two, is not divulged. It is not difficult to imagine, though, that the men interviewed by Smith were experiencing a range of emotions. These would comprise reactions to their childbirth education, to their experience of the birth and to their ongoing adjustment to fatherhood.

The informants, however, were not invariably negative about their experiences of childbirth education. The fathers appreciated any acknowledgement of the role they sought to perform and any guidelines about the help they could provide during labour. The material taught about life with the new baby which was most appreciated was that which was practical, in terms of helpful tips, and balanced without too much emphasis on the negative aspects. To illustrate this latter point, one father, Dave, reported:

> There was nothing really upbeat about being a parent . . . [the midwife] was slightly negative about it. She rushed through it. She didn't say any plus things about being a parent and it was all about sleepless nights.
> (Smith, 1999a: 25)

As well as criticisms of the negativity and the unreality of the classes, their relevance was also questioned. The issue of relevance, however, was related more to the ability (i.e. 'skills, awareness, understanding') of the teacher. The fathers considered that the quality of the teaching was crucial (1999c: 468). Criticisms of the classes' relevance are summarised in the comment by Rob who described himself as having been 'an observer at a class for women' (1999a: 25). It is necessary to question whether this reaction, as in the Finnish study mentioned above, constitutes a case of 'shooting the messenger'.

The issue of the relevance of the material, which was clearly a major problem for the fathers, deserves attention. The fathers were very clear about what they did not want to be taught; these were matters of fact or reality. What the fathers appear to have been seeking were the emotional factors and the positive side of the experience. It may be that this is a very selective choice of information and it hardly constitutes 'the whole birth thing' which they sought, as mentioned above.

The rationale for this selectivity may be associated with the man's limited exposure to the informal knowledge, or 'old wives' tales about childbearing, which is acquired by his partner over years of woman-to-woman contact. It may be that the man expected the classes to compensate for this long-standing deficiency. His woman partner, on the other hand, may have had too much of this 'informal knowledge' and came to the classes in search of up-to-date, in-depth information. Thus the agendas of the two partners, or their reasons for attending childbirth education, may be diametrically opposed.

The differing needs of the male and female partners are exemplified in the limited attention, according to Smith's sample, given in the classes to the postnatal events. The woman is likely to be unconcerned about this limitation, since she knows that she will have mothers, neighbours and friends to help her at that crucial time. The woman's major need is for information about the labour, when she is effectively on her own.

The recommendations arising out of Smith's study (1999a: 25) suggest that the classes should be matched to the man's expectations of his experience of the birth and the fatherhood which follows it. This matching may be difficult as, apart from the reality or otherwise of the man's expectations, they are bound to be individual, and may not even be conscious, recognised or articulated.

The underlying problem of childbirth education for a man is his difficulty in conceiving of the wide range of healthy experiences which constitute physiological uncomplicated childbirth. There may, similarly, be difficulty in comprehending the huge variation in emotional inputs and reactions to child-birth. It may be that a man views childbearing in a Cartesian or mechanistic way. This may be comparable to their medical brothers, with assumptions of specific inputs and outputs, without recognising or acknowledging the vast human variability. The same observation applies to the experience of life with a newborn baby. There may be difficulty in understanding how, due to a wide range of known, unknown and unknowable factors, the first weeks, months and years vary hugely in their congeniality.

One of the criticisms which has been levelled at childbirth education is summarised by Nolan as the view of the father as 'mother's little helper' (1998: 148). In spite of such critical recognition, the focus which persists is predominantly on the father as one of the supporters for the woman in labour. As a result, the material concentrates on teaching him how to undertake this role. These criticisms lead into a crucial examination of the role of the father in childbearing.

The father's role

As indicated above, uncertainty about what role the father takes during the birth and afterwards is likely to cause difficulty in childbirth education.

The role at a certain time

There is one particular point where the problem becomes critical and this was quite serendipitously identified in a small study by Koppel and Kaiser (2001). These researchers planned a qualitative study to examine the experience of the father in the neonatal intensive care unit (NICU). A sample of eighteen fathers of newborn babies was successfully recruited. The fathers were keen to talk to the researcher but, unfortunately for the research design, did not wish to talk about their experience of being a father in an NICU.

The data which emerged hinged on the birth of the baby, which for most of the informants was by caesarean operation under general anaesthesia. Of the eighteen births, seventeen were by caesarean. Four of these fathers were present at the birth. Of the remaining thirteen, ten (77 per cent) of the fathers were shocked to find that they were prevented from being with their partner during the birth. The reason given to these men was that the caesarean was being performed under a general anaesthetic. These fathers' exclusion was in spite of 'heated debates and/or desperate pleas' (2001: 250). Thus, the situation arises of the father ordinarily being strenuously encouraged to accompany his partner at the birth. When his presence would later be most helpful, though (that is, when she is not conscious), his presence is effectively vetoed. The paradoxical nature of this scenario has been noted previously by Oakley and Richards (1990) and in Chapter 4, pp. 88–90, this volume.

Koppel and Kaiser (2001) focus on the fathers' emotional reactions to their exclusion, hence the highly graphic title of the paper 'Fathers at the end of their rope'. This title is a more emotive translation of the rather British 'end of the tether'. The apparent change in the direction of the rope from horizontal to vertical carries sinister allusions. As well as the fathers being appropriately distraught, they complained vehemently about the lack of information. For this reason their disenchantment was aggravated by their anxiety about their partner and the baby. Although these authors question why these fathers were not permitted to be present at the birth, they omit to relate this to the role of the father in childbearing. Thus the question remains unasked: 'What is the father's role that he is able to perform at a caesarean with epidural anaesthesia that he can't perform when a general anaesthetic is used?'

Koppel and Kaiser's small but important research project leads into a crucial examination of the precise nature of the father's role in childbearing. It is only when his role is fully understood that the father will be able to be assured of a satisfactory and satisfying experience of the birth of the couple's child.

The father's general role

The man's role was mentioned briefly when, in the early chapters of this book, I sought to address the reality, or practical aspects, of the man's involvement with childbearing (Chapter 3, p. 78). To do this, I used anecdotes to trace the man's entry into the birthing room and research to explore his reaction to finding himself there. Although my discussion concentrated on the more concrete aspects of his situation, I did refer to the invaluable work by Draper (1997) which spans the divide between the theoretical aspects of his presence and its application. Having previously examined the practice in the birthing room and the input of childbirth education earlier in this chapter, I move on now to focus on the more theoretical aspects of the man's situation. The intention is that this material will provide insights into how the midwife may ameliorate, or even remedy, the problems which have been shown to be inherent in the man's involvement in childbearing generally and his presence in the birthing room in particular.

A useful contribution to our understanding of the man's position is found in the research work by Chapman (1992). Using grounded theory methodology, she sought to generate a theoretical framework which would illuminate the man's experience of labour and birth. Observations in the labour room and interviews within four weeks of the birth led her to an understanding of the helical relationship between the three major variables. These are the expectations of the woman, the expectations of her partner and the progress of the labour. As a result of this helix, she proposes that the man may adopt one of three possible roles at any given time:

- *The coach* – who provides instruction
- *The team mate* – who provides support
- *The witness* – who is present.

The demands of these three roles are clearly very different in terms of the man's emotional, psychological and physical involvement with the woman and her labour. A hierarchical relationship may be seen to exist between the three roles, with the coach being the most actively involved and the witness the least. Chapman found that which of these three roles the man assumes at any given time is affected by four major 'conditions'. She maintains that these 'conditions' relate to:

1   his expectations
2   the couple's relationship
3   the guidance he is offered
4   the state of his health.

These 'conditions' are seriously problematical, since the first two are virtually unknowable by the couple and even less knowable by outsiders. For this reason, their contribution in practice should be disregarded.

The third 'condition', however, may be of more value because it involves the indications of what activity is needed. These indications comprise the cues given by his partner, such as asking for iced water either verbally or non-verbally. Alternatively the cues may be the more explicit instructions by the birth attendant, such as to mobilise more actively or to adopt a different posture. On the basis of such an active input, Chapman suggests that the man feels involved and is able to maintain his role. This means that his position on the hierarchy of roles is secure and he does not begin to slip down the hierarchy and risk becoming less satisfied.

The work of Chapman may be criticised for its mechanistic approach to the man's role, but in spite of this she demonstrates some valuable issues. First is the recognition of the three roles which the man may seek to adopt, although these roles should be recognised as points on a continuum rather than as discrete entities. Probably more important, though, is the way Chapman shows the dynamic nature of the father's role. His role is in no way a static phenomenon. She indicates the immense scope for variation in role even within one individual father in one labour. Chapman also suggests the way that these variations are likely to be affected by a wide range of internal and external phenomena. These variations are reflected in fluctuations in his position on the hierarchy of roles. It would be wrong to imply that any value judgement is present in this hierarchy, although the father's perception may be a different matter.

The fourth of the 'conditions' which Chapman lists is the state of the man's health. This may appear to be of minimal consequence once it is realised that the stereotype of the father fainting in the labour room is almost unheard of (in my experience it is medical students who are infinitely more likely to keel over). Research, however, indicates otherwise.

Having recognised some of the problems for the father attending the birth, Johnson (2002a) sought to begin to correct the deficiency in the literature focusing on the father. He prepared for a study of the father's stress, associated with pressure on him to attend the birth, and his unfulfilled expectations. Johnson suggests that one of the factors which aggravates the man's stress is that he is a witness to his partner's pain, which he is quite impotent to remedy (see Chapter 4, pp. 93–5, this volume). This researcher used quantitative measures to assess the fifty-three men's experience of childbearing. The Impact of Events Scale (IES) was used to measure the men's stress levels during pregnancy, at the time of the birth and again when the baby was 6 weeks old.

In this study certain contradictions relating to the father's role at the birth were identified and endorsed. The first was the problem, mentioned above, of the woman experiencing pain when the man was not in any position to help her by relieving it. The second major contradiction impinging on the man's role is found in the vast discrepancy between his expectations of the experience and the reality of the birth. During pregnancy a large majority of the men (n = 34; 83 per cent) articulated their expectations of being able to assume an active role in their partner's labour. Most of the men (n = 39; 73.6 per cent) saw their role as to provide support for their partner, whereas a much smaller proportion were only looking forward to bonding with the baby. The relatively small number (n = 6; 11 per cent), who did not know why they were going to be present, is particularly disconcerting. Even these fairly modest expectations, however, remained unfulfilled. A majority (n = 23; 53.7 per cent) of the men considered themselves to have been unable to even be supportive. For an even higher number, though, their largely negative feelings were summarised by the 56 per cent (n = 23) whose overall feelings were reflected in the words of one of the fathers who felt that he had been 'in the way' (Johnson, 2002a: 178).

Another disconcerting finding, which may not be unrelated to the one mentioned above, is the widespread (n = 25; 61 per cent) perception among the men that they were forced to be present at the birth. In view of the frequent occurrence of this perception, it may be surprising that so few of the men did not know why they were present. When the men were asked about the source of this pressure or coercion to attend, they reported that (in descending order of frequency) it came from the hospital staff, their partners, their family and their friends. The order of this pressure may be surprising, but is probably explained by the fact that *any* pressure from health care providers is unacceptable. In a culture where attendance at the birth is the norm, however, pressure from the remaining sources may pass unremarked. Irrespective of the validity of this finding, it is disturbing that Johnson found that measured stress was highest among the men who perceived some degree of coercion to be present.

On the basis of his findings, Johnson was able to draw certain conclusions about the man's childbirth education. One of these points is reminiscent of the 'messenger-shooting' criticisms mentioned above (see pp. 163–6). The fathers contend that they would have been more likely to learn from their childbirth education if their teacher had been of the same gender:

> I know at the classes the midwife bangs on about stuff, but it's not like a bloke explaining what it was like for them, and when they do say, what they say is often the crap they are supposed to, rather than the reality.
> (Johnson, 2002a: 177)

This observation is advanced in spite of the finding, by Smith (1999a, 1999b, 1999c), that childbirth education by a midwife who is a male did not improve the fathers' learning or their experience. Johnson builds on these comments by suggesting that what the men actually need is explanations from a man who is a father. This requirement comes round to the preference for an experienced father who is willing and able to share his real experience, rather than the 'sanitized version' (2002a: 1977), which Johnson maintains is the norm among male peers. These recommendations serve to ignore the huge variation, mentioned above, in healthy childbearing experiences. Thus, even if the father-to-be were to be given an 'unsanitised version', it might well be of little or no value if his own experience proved to be different. A suggestion which may be appropriate in assisting the father may be found in the literature on child/siblings attending the birth (Jonquil, 1993). It is recommended that a dedicated companion should be 'there' for the child at the birth, to give explanations and only to attend to all of the child's needs. While the presence of yet another person in the birthing room may be far from welcome, this person might effectively facilitate a more satisfactory role for the man and, hence, be of indirect assistance to the woman. In cultures where the 'doula' is unnecessary due to the tradition of midwifery care, the doula could thus be gainfully employed (Mander, 2001a).

The men's unpreparedness for the birth appears, like the men interviewed by Smith (1999a, see above), to have engendered considerable emotional tension. This is clear from the men's words:

> I was shocked by what she went through . . . I knew it would hurt her . . . but it eats in to you as the time goes on – especially as you can't help her – not really.
>
> (Ben, in Johnson, 2002b: 176)

> The pain was terrible to watch, worse than last time.
>
> (Francis, in ibid.)

Thus, on the basis of his findings, Johnson (2002b) appears to have highlighted the paradoxical weakness of childbirth education in preparing the man to accompany his partner at the birth. Johnson emphasises the way in which the father perceives that he has not been well prepared in his role as the 'coach' and, as if this shortcoming were not sufficient, neither is he prepared for the full impact of his experience of birth (2002b: 180).

In view of this paradox, Johnson's question 'Are men prepared for their role?' (2002b: 176) has a rhetorical ring. The only possible reply seems to be 'How can they be?' This response is due to a number of confounding factors.

Confounding factors

The first confounding factor is the paradox mentioned above.

The second is another contrast between the usual pattern of the couple's life and the situation they are required to face in labour. Johnson shows the reader that the man is in a particularly vulnerable position because his usual source of support – his female partner – has been removed. What is more, his female partner is not only not supporting him, she is in urgent and desperate need of an intensity of support which he was unaware even existed, let alone ever provided.

The third confounding factor is the problems relating to the role. Each man brings his own expectations, which are somewhere on the continuum described by Chapman (above). These expectations are individual and may be unconscious, unrecognised and unarticulated. They also change dynamically as the labour progresses. As well as the man's largely intangible expectations, there are differing expectations among the others who may be involved. Johnson (2002a: 181) identifies the differing expectations of the man's role among 'obstetricians, midwives, parturients and expectant fathers'. He goes on to state that these expectations need to be more fully explored.

Thus a number of paradoxes arise out of Johnson's research. The main message which he drew from his study, however, is found in the link between coercion on the father to be present, causing him to be stressed. It could be that the linking factor between these two phenomena may be found in the futility which so many men in his sample articulated.

Draper (1997) regards this scenario as a self-fulfilling prophecy comprising low expectations among staff and plummeting self-confidence in the men (see Chapter 4, p. 72, this volume). This explanation is unrealistically simplistic, bearing in mind the variations in all of the individuals and phenomena involved in the process of childbirth.

Helping the medical practitioner

The help available to the medical practitioner may be considered only in terms of that which exists to maintain or reinforce the existing medical domination of health care. This may not, in the long term, be helpful to the medical practitioner or to those for whom he is intended to provide a service. In this section, therefore, I address the remedial action which may facilitate the colossal changes needed to benefit the medical fraternity and the consumer.

In the context of childbearing, the major problems for the medical practitioner are those which arose out of the analysis in Chapter 4 (see pp. 92–6), and which may be summarised as follows:

- Assumption of the pathological nature of childbearing
- Lack of understanding of the physiological nature of labour pain
- Anachronistic mechanistic or Cartesian attitudes to childbearing
- Hospitalisation of birth for educational and/or research purposes
- Defensive attitudes leading to interventive practice
- Reluctance to practise evidence-based, or even research-based, medicine.

While these problems constitute the culture of medicine, their source is difficult to identify. The result, however, is readily apparent in the medicalisation of childbearing. The continuation of these problems, though, is self-perpetuating in the hothouse atmosphere which is medical education. The pathologically narrow focus of medical education is notorious (Scully, 1994). There is a long overdue need for the winds of change to be blown through medical education. The aim of this fumigation would be to expose medical students to ideas other than those ingrained by centuries of dogma. Teaching would be by health care personnel of other disciplines and by academics from outwith health care. This revolution would introduce fresh ideas and ways of thinking and learning. This would include gaining under-standing from clients and patients (Mander, 1988, 1989), from other health care professionals and from other learners.

A major development which is moving in the direction of this transfor-mation of medical education is the movement which is becoming known as 'multiprofessional education'. Unfortunately, this term is subject to mis-interpretation, since the English National Board defined it as involving only 'non-medical health care students' (2001: 5). This form of shared learning is subject to considerable variations in terminology as well as definition. The term 'interprofessional education' may be preferable because it indicates the profound engagement of the professional groups with each other (Barr and Waterton, 1996). Because it is less widely used, though, I am reluctant to use this term. Since multiprofessional education was first mooted it has engendered misgivings, particularly among medical practitioners (Atkins, 1998). There have long been concerns relating to loss of professional identity, which Atkins suggests would best be addressed by confidence-building activities and the recognition of unique professional traditions. In those settings where multiprofessional education has begun to be introduced (Howe *et al.*, 2002), the process has given rise to some discomfort. Howe and her colleagues found that medical students were reluctant to take seriously the non-clinical material, and other 'stakeholders' and service users found that medical students tended towards arrogance. This behaviour was attributed to earlier unfortunate experiences in other learning situations.

Medicine, not surprisingly, considers that it has most to lose and least to gain from the introduction of multiprofessional education. For this reason, medicine has argued most strongly against its introduction (Campbell and Johnston, 1999; Finch, 2000). While specific clinical areas have been intro-duced to facilitate multiprofessional education (Reeves *et al.*, 2002; Wahlstrom *et al.*, 1997), this innovative practice may be too late, since it may follow the acquisition of negative stereotypes by the learner (Leaviss, 2000). Sternas and colleagues (1999) argue that collaborative behaviour must be learned at a much earlier stage in their education by students, certainly before any other disadvantageous attitudes are acquired. In this way, through learn-ing to understand and respect each other's roles, those who are involved with the care of the childbearing woman and her partner may acquire sufficient confidence in their own functioning to be able to dispense with the professional coping strategies listed above.

Conclusion

The research and other literature shows that a number of strategies have been adopted to ameliorate the position of the man in the childbearing situation. The father and the medical practitioner have and are being subjected to a variety of educational and other interventions which are intended to be helpful to them. In this chapter, the literature has shown that these strategies have so far met with little, if any, success.

The research literature has shown very clearly the emotional reaction of the father to his experience of being present at the birth. This reaction has featured shock and barely suppressed anger. A tendency has emerged which involves the more articulate father blaming the system, which he feels has let him down. This blame may be attributed to the hospital, the childbirth education classes, his employment or to the personnel of the operating theatre. Because the studies involved tended to be qualitative, it may be necessary to question whether these findings reflect the experience of the majority of fathers. No literature has been identified which suggests that these qualitative studies' findings are anything but accurate.

Thus the many attempts by both researchers and practitioners to resolve the problems associated with men's involvement in childbearing have not been successful. On the basis of my reading of the literature, I suggest that these enlightened and well-meaning attempts to improve the man's position are doomed to failure. The reason for this is that one crucially important question still remains to be answered. This question, which is applied to both male attendants and to the father, relates to the rationale for the man's involvement in childbearing and to who is the intended beneficiary of his presence. In more precise terms, the role of the father in particular has still to be clearly defined. The literature used in this book indicates that there is no clear definition of his role and that there is massive uncertainty. This absence of role definition results in a number of paradoxes and contradictions being faced by the father when he is least able to confront them.

In order to clarify these issues, it is necessary to ask certain fundamental questions about the role of the father and the role of the medical practitioner. These questions will be formulated in Chapter 9.

Conclusion

Through the medium of this book, I have made an attempt to explore and deconstruct a curiously modern phenomenon. This modern curiosity is the involvement of the man in the latter stages of the process of childbearing. The participation of a man in the early stages, by which I mean at the conception, is widely accepted as a fact of life. With the advent of assisted reproduction techniques, however, even this role may be undergoing a process of change.

It may be that this book will be interpreted by some as yet another example of a man-bashing tirade. If this is the perception of some who read it, I regard that as unfortunate. To produce such a tirade is certainly not my intention. In the preparation of this book, I have intended throughout to examine as objectively as possible the relevant research literature. On the occasions when those sources do not exist, I have sought to use other literature. Adopting as academic an orientation as possible, I have strenuously avoided a selective approach to the literature. Such selection obviously would have had the effect of introducing some personal bias. Even after using the most efficient searching techniques, though, it is possible that some of the existing literature has been overlooked. If this is the case, it is in no way deliberate.

Context

Before endeavouring, in this concluding chapter, to sum up the arguments which have emerged from this scrutiny of men's contribution to childbearing, a brief recap of the context may be helpful. The first point which should be borne in mind is the *significance of childbearing*. As well as its health, personal and demographic implications, its sociological importance needs to be re-emphasised. Childbearing represents a reflection of many aspects of the culture in which it happens. This is a reflection which applies regardless of whether the process is socially determined, domestically oriented or medically dominated. As well as its broad societal significance, childbearing is also a rite of passage for the parents as individuals and, possibly, as a couple. While they are entering motherhood and fatherhood, the woman and man respectively achieve considerably more than this. The couple may have been physically mature for varying periods at the time of the birth. It is, however, the fact of becoming parents that, in the eyes of many, metamorphoses them into real adults. Thus childbearing facilitates entry into the world of the adult, complete with all of its rights as well as responsibilities and obligations.

The second contextual point to bear in mind is the *extent of the change* represented by the entry of the man into the healthy childbearing scenario. I have shown that prior to the entrance of the man-midwife, which began with the Chamberlen dynasty at the close of the sixteenth century, men were barred from the birth of a live baby. As well as being excluded by the women attendants, the men sought to exclude themselves by creating the concept known as pollution. Around this concept grew a theoretical edifice of taboos. These prohibitions have been incorporated into the major world religions and have permitted men to retain a large measure of control over women's childbearing activities, in spite of being physically remote from such events. Thus the man has chosen to reverse this mutually determined exclusion. As a birth attendant, the man has assumed variably direct control over childbearing. This has happened to the extent that in some countries, such as those in North America, the man has at times sought, or even managed, to totally exclude the traditional female carer.

As well as the change for the carer, the role of the husband or partner has undergone a revolutionary change. While the partner has also traditionally been excluded from the process of childbearing, this situation was reversed in the latter part of the twentieth century. The result is that, together with his social contemporaries, the attendants who formerly barred his entry are now encouraging him to be involved, to the point of compelling his participation. This encouragement has been shown by research to have become something of a carrot which is stick shaped. The man's reaction to his involvement may be said to be 'not unmixed'.

Emergent themes

Having reflected briefly on the context of the man's presence, it is now necessary to draw together the major themes which have emerged in this analysis of the current position of the man in childbearing.

Problems – the evidence

The first and most pervasive theme to emerge from the material which has been examined in this book is that men have problems with childbearing. These problems have been shown to manifest themselves in a number of ways.

The first evidence is the existence of an alteration in the man's behaviour and functioning. These alterations have become recognised as the various forms of *couvade*. This behavioural manifestation has been interpreted in a number of ways; these include couvade as a form of sympathy with his partner, as a visible expression of his changing role and as a plea for help in coming to terms with the momentous changes in his life and relationships.

Further evidence of the man's difficulty with childbearing is to be found in the unequivocal data on the increased incidence of *domestic violence* in association with pregnancy and the puerperium. That the man perceives his partner's developing relationship with the fetus and baby as a threat to his controlling power over the couple's relationship is a persuasive explanation of this form of abuse.

The wealth of data on the man's impressions of his *experience of the birth* constitutes the third example of his difficulties with childbearing. It has been shown that, while the electronic media in particular present a strongly favourable picture of this experience, the research data clearly demonstrate his less positive reactions to being present at the birth. The reasons for these reactions are not entirely clear. They may however be associated with the uncertainty as to his role or his inability to influence the experience which he and his partner are facing.

The last of the manifestations of the man's problems with childbearing may be found in the practice of the *medical profession*. This difficulty is demonstrated by the medical attendant's inability to recognise childbearing as the healthy, physiological process which it almost invariably is. This may be due to the nature of medical education or perhaps because of the masculine orientation of the medical profession. Medical practitioners are unable to await the healthy outcome which would be the result of the vast majority of unmedicalised childbearing experiences. Instead of this 'attendance', the compulsion to control physiological processes has been demonstrated since a man first entered the healthy birthing room. Initially this control was through the introduction of the obstetric forceps. The forceps, however, were succeeded by a range of instruments, drugs, machines and surgical operations which have been intended to shorten the process of childbearing.

Conspiracy theory

These problems tend not to be discussed. In the case of our medical brothers this is because they are not seen as problems, but as opportunities for personal and/or professional development. In the case of the man who is a partner, though, his situation is quite different. Prior to the birth the father is led to anticipate an experience which, though challenging, is unlikely to be beyond his personal coping resources. He anticipates that he will be able to draw on the skills which he has developed as a man and which he has learned during childbirth education. This is what he has come to expect and nobody has informed him otherwise. His confidence is likely to have been boosted by what he has learned about the scientific or measurable aspects of childbearing. The principles of the functioning of the childbearing human body, his medical brothers will have assured him in a Cartesian way, are not really very different from the functioning of the internal combustion engine.

The man's confident expectations apply to both the labour and birth as well as to the early days, weeks and months of fatherhood. The skills which he anticipates using are essentially his ability to be able to protect his partner from any adverse experiences and, if that protection is not wholly effective, to be able to resolve or 'fix' the adversity. The man realises very quickly, though, that the nature of labour is qualitatively and quantitatively different from anything for which he had prepared himself. He soon finds himself out of his depth as well as out of place.

The man's misgivings and feelings of unpreparedness do not end with the birth. The arrival of the new baby into his life and into his relationship changes that life and that relationship utterly. In addition, this new situation arouses feelings of a depth and intensity which were previously quite unknown to him. It is at this time that the man begins to question why he had not been told that this situation and these feelings would develop. He eventually comes to realise that there exists a conspiracy of silence among men. To admit that fatherhood is anything other than a delightfully satisfying experience would reflect adversely on his manhood. Such an admission would also cause him to lose face with his partner, his family and, possibly most importantly, his contemporaries. This cultural taboo on the man's self-revelation emerges clearly in Chapter 7 (see pp. 143–7). In this way the conspiracy of silence is perpetuated.

Self-fulfilling prophecies

It may be regarded as unfortunate that in terms of his expectations the man is not functioning on a level playing field. The odds would appear to be stacked against him in a number of ways. Thus there are certain self-fulfilling prophecies operating, although he is unaware of their existence. In chronological terms the first of these is encountered during his partner's labour and was identified by Draper (1997; see Chapter 4, p. 82 above). She found that the labour ward staff influence the father's expectations of his role and, by diminishing those expectations and belittling that role, effectively create a self-fulfilling prophecy. Although, as mentioned above, his expectations are initially high, the staff lower his expectations of what the father is able and permitted to contribute during the labour and birth. In this way, his feelings of being out of his depth and out of place are aggravated when he is made to feel totally incompetent.

Another self-fulfilling prophecy which further threatens his self-esteem is likely to materialise later in his experience of fatherhood. It relates to his partner breast-feeding their baby. In the general, and entirely appropriate, enthusiasm to promote breast-feeding, the hurdles faced by the mother and father tend to be minimised, if not ignored. Following their research Jordan and Wall (1990; see Chapter 5, pp. 106–8 above) argue that both parents should be prepared more realistically for their role. This role would feature the overwhelming commitment of the mother and the cruel marginality of the father. Such realistic preparation would present a dismal picture with the potential to become a self-fulfilling prophecy if the couple are not taught how to overcome these hurdles.

The unholy alliance

An overarching theme which has emerged already (see Chapter 4, pp. 97–8) is the concept of the unholy alliance. This may, however, apply more generally than in the context of the birth. The underlying factors which lead to the manifestation of this phenomenon relate to the behaviour of the two groups of men in the childbearing scenario. On the one hand there is the father, feeling out of his depth and out of place. On the other hand are the medical attendants seeking opportunities to practise their professional obstetric skills by intervening in the woman's childbearing process. The two groups come to recognise in each other, not just a shared gender orientation or a kindred spirit. Each finds an ally who will help the other to resolve the differently difficult situation in which he finds himself. Thus, together they identify a common agenda which happens by chance to meet the needs of both groups. In effect, this alliance is a common solution to very different problems.

The situation in which this is most readily apparent and which has been mentioned already (Chapter 4, pp. 97–8) is in the context of the *control of labour pain*. This happens when the father is unable to cope with being impotent to resolve the pain of the woman in labour. The medical practitioner offers his pharmacological solution, such as an epidural analgesia, which allows a cascade of medical interventions and at the same time resolves the father's feelings of impotence.

Another, not unrelated, manifestation of the unholy alliance would be found in the woman whose partograph shows that the progress of her labour has fallen below the action line. In such a situation, even though the mother and fetus are not physically distressed, the medical practitioner would diagnose *prolonged labour* or even 'failure to progress'. The woman could be persuaded to agree to a caesarean by being presented with the unarguable fact that she is tired. The medical practitioner would have the opportunity to practise his surgical skills, as well as dealing with the surgical complications and the likelihood of a 'secondary caesarean' in any future pregnancies. The father would be relieved, because his uncertainty about the duration of labour would be brought to an end by this untimely intervention.

A further example of the unholy alliance may be found in the much earlier days of the woman's pregnancy. This is when the couple are given the opportunity to 'meet' their baby through the medium of a routine *ultrasound scan*. The usual rationale is that the early scan provides an accurate gestational asessment, yet in reality a number of other agendas are operating. To the father he is being given an intimate insight into the presence of the baby which has previously been denied to him. Further, he has scientific evidence of a pregnancy which had previously been his partner's unique experience. To the medical practitioner, however, he is searching for fetal 'anomalies' which present an opportunity to intervene in this otherwise healthy pregnancy. Thus, for their diametrically opposed reasons, the father and the medical practitioner are keen that the scan is undertaken. The mother, meanwhile, has the opportunity to see a baby with whom she is already intimately acquainted and, as a result, has her confidence in her own innate knowledge of the baby effectively demolished.

The questions

A number of crucial questions emerge out of this analysis of the man's input into the healthy childbearing process.

What are the benefits?

The modern system of health care requires that any intervention needs to be justified. This means that any activity should be shown to be effective, that is, successful in achieving its aims. Thus it is necessary to examine the man's involvement in terms of it being something other than 'nice' or 'traditional'. In a health care system which aspires, and perhaps even claims, to being evidence-based, these totally unevaluated interventions are paradoxical. Further, if there is even a slim possibility that these men's involvement may be anything other than beneficial, this needs to be addressed.

Who benefits?

If there is an assumption that there are benefits, it is necessary to ascertain to whom they accrue. Are the benefits to:

- The partner
- The medical practitioner
- The woman
- The baby?

My analysis earlier in this chapter suggests that the partner certainly does not benefit. The woman appears to be at risk of certain potentially iatrogenic interventions. This latter risk applies to a lesser extent to the baby.

What is the evidence that medical involvement improves outcomes?

In view of the implicit suggestion in the answer to the second question that the medical practitioner is the only beneficiary, the evidence that his contribution affects and improves outcomes should be made clear. Research which has sought to investigate the roles of the various providers has invariably suffered from the inevitable controlling influence of medical practitioners in drawing up the research protocols. This has not facilitated objectivity. The principles of the randomised controlled trial (RCT), regarded as the gold standard in medical research, need to be applied to the involvement of the medical practitioner in healthy childbearing.

Is there a role for the man as a partner? If so, what is the nature of that role?

Many of the difficulties experienced by the partner in the context of child-bearing, as well as the justification problem (see above), appear to relate to the uncertain nature of his role. In Chapter 8 this question began to emerge (pp. 173–4). While the woman has been shown to value her partner's presence, it is necessary to question whether this is sufficient justification for his involvement in view of the evidence of his experience.

An open debate about the partner and his contribution is essential. It may be that the couple are encouraged to contemplate whether, for them, his involvement will be neither helpful nor necessary. Such a situation would permit an openness which is currently not acceptable. If the couple decide that the father should be involved, they may need to be assisted to decide the nature of his role. Further, they may consider how that role will develop in the event of the labour, birth and early child care progressing along more (or less) expected lines. If the father is ever to achieve a satisfying and satisfactory experience in the childbearing scenario, the fundamental question of the nature of his role, if any, requires to be answered.

References

About (2002) Couvade: sympathetic pregnancy http://pregnancy.about.com/library/weekly/aa033197.htm. Accessed 24 January.

Ahern, E.M. (1978) The power and pollution of Chinese women (pp. 269–90), in A.P. Wolf (ed.) *Studies in Chinese Society*. Stanford, CA: Stanford University Press.

Arney, W.R. (1982) *Power and the Profession of Obstetrics*. Chicago, IL: University of Chicago Press.

Atkins, J. (1998) Tribalism loss and grief issues for multiprofessional education. *Journal of Interprofessional Care* 12 (3): 303–7.

Aveling, J.H. (1882) *The Chamberlens and the Midwifery Forceps: Memorials of the Family and an Essay on the Invention of the Instrument*. London: J. & A. Churchill.

Backwell, J. (1977) Husband in the labour ward. *Midwives Chronicle* November: 270–2.

Bahl, K. (1996) Perspectives. Towards equality . . . the Equal Opportunities Commission's 20th anniversary. *Nursing Standard* 10 (27): 19.

Barbour, R. (1990) Fathers: a new consumer group (ch. 11, p. 202), in J. Garcia, R. Kilpatrick and M. Richards (eds) *The Politics of Maternity Care*. Oxford: Clarendon Press.

Barclay, L. and Lupton, D. (1999) The experiences of new fatherhood: a socio-cultural analysis. *Journal of Advanced Nursing* 29 (4): 1013–20.

Barclay, L., Andre, C.A. and Glover, P.A. (1989) Women's business: the challenge of childbirth. *Midwifery* 5 (3): 122–33.

Bar-On, R. (1997) *Bar-On Emotional Quotient Inventory: A Measure of Emotional Intelligence*. Technical Manual. Toronto: Multi-Health Systems.

Barr, H. and Waterton, S. (1996) *Interprofessional Education in Health and Social Care in the United Kingdom*. London: CAIPE.

Barr, R. (1988) A long day's journey into life . . . a father's account of the birth of his first child. *Midwives Chronicle* 101 (1208): 271–2.

Bartels, R. (1999) Experience of childbirth from the father's perspective. *British Journal of Midwifery* 7 (11): 681–3.

Bates, C. (1997) Care in normal labour: a feminist perspective (ch. 9, p. 127), in J. Alexander, V. Levy and C. Roth (eds) *Midwifery Practice*. Core Topics 2. London: Macmillan.

Beardshaw, T. (2001) Supporting the role of fathers around the time of birth. *MIDIRS* 11 (4): 476–9.

Beauchamp, T.L. and Childress, J.F. (1994) *Principles of Biomedical Ethics* (4th edn). New York/Oxford: Oxford University Press.

Beckmann, C.A., Van Mullem, C., Beckmann, C.R. and Broekhuizen, F.F. (1997) Interpreting fetal heart rate tracings. Is there a difference between labor and delivery nurses and obstetricians? *Journal of Reproductive Medicine* 42(10): 647–50.

Bedford, V.A. and Johnson, N. (1988) The role of the father. *Midwifery* 4 (4): 190–5.

Beech, B. (1996) Court ordered caesareans – a hidden abuse. *AIMS Journal* 8 (3): 1–4.

Beech B. and Thomas, P. (2001) 40 years ago . . . men in the labour wards. *AIMS Journal* 12 (4): 7–8.

Beech, B. and Robinson, J. (1996) *Ultrasound? Unsound AIMS.* London: Association for Improvements in Maternity Services.

Bennett, A., Hewson, B., Booker, E. and Holliday, S. (1985) Antenatal preparation and labor support in relation to birth outcomes. *Birth* 12: 9–16.

Bertola, C. and Drakich, J. (1995) The father's rights movement ch. 12, in W. Marsiglio (ed.) *Fatherhood: Contemporary Theory, Research and Social Policy.* Thousand Oaks, CA: Sage.

Bertsch T.D., Nagashima-Whalen, L., Dykeman, S., Kennell, J. and McGrath, S. (1990) Labor support by first time fathers. *Journal of Psychosomatic Obstetrics and Gynaecology* 11: 251–60.

Bettelheim, B. (1954) *Symbolic Wounds.* Glencoe, IL: Free Press.

Beutel, M., Willner, H., Deckardt, R., Von Rad, M. and Weiner, H. (1996) Similarities and differences in couples' grief reactions following a miscarriage: results from a longitudinal study. *Journal of Psychosomatic Research* 4 (3): 245–253.

Bewley, C. (2002a) Fact or fallacy? Domestic violence in pregnancy: an overview. *MIDIRS Midwifery Digest* 12 (Supp 2): S3–S5.

Bewley, C. (2002b) Personal communication.

Bewley, C. and Gibbs, A. (2000) Domestic violence and pregnancy: a midwifery issue (ch. 7), in J. Alexander, C. Roth and V. Levy (eds) *Midwifery Practice.* Core Topics 3. London: Macmillan.

Bewley, C. and Gibbs, A. (2001) Domestic abuse and pregnancy: writing policies and protocols. *MIDIRS Midwifery Digest* 11 (2): 183–7.

Bounty UK Ltd (2003) http://www.bounty.com/. Accessed April.

Bourne, S. (1968) The psychological effects of stillbirth on women and their doctors. *Journal of Royal College of General Practitioners* 16: 103–12.

Bowlby, J. (1958) The nature of the child's tie to his mother. *International Journal of Psychoanalysis* 30: 350.

Boyle, F.M. (1997) *Mothers Bereaved by Stillbirth, Neonatal Death or Sudden Infant Death Syndrome.* Aldershot: Ashgate.

Brannen, J. and Moss, P. (1988) *New Mothers at Work: Employment and Childcare.* London: Unwin.

Bricker, L., Garcia, J., Henderson, J., Mugford, M., Neilson, J., Roberts, T. and Martin, M-A. (2000) Ultrasound screening in pregnancy: a systematic review of the clinical effectiveness, cost-effectiveness and women's views. *Health Technology Assessment* 4 (16): http://www.hta.nhsweb.nhs.uk/execsumm/summ416.htm.

Bronfenbrenner, U. (1961) Some familial antecedents of responsibility and leadership in adolescents, in L. Petrullo and B. M. Bass (eds) *Leadership and Interpersonal Behavior.* New York: Holt, Rinehart & Winston.

Brown, A. (1982) Fathers in the labour ward (ch. 7, p. 104), in L. McKee and M. O'Brien (eds) *The Father Figure*. London: Tavistock.

Brownlee, M., Mackintosh, C.L., Wallace, E.M., Johnstone, F.D. and Murphy-Black, F.D. (1996) A survey of interprofessional communication in a labour suite. *British Journal of Midwifery* 4 (9): 492–5.

Bryson, V. (1999) Patriarchy: a concept too useful to lose? The concept of patriarchy: still a useful concept? University of Huddersfield: www.psa.ac.uk/cps/1999/bryson.pdf. Accessed 10 July 2003.

Burdette Saunders, R. (1999) Nursing care during pregnancy (ch. 10, p. 206), in D. Lowdermilk, S.E. Perry and I.M. Bobak (eds) *Maternity Nursing* (5th edn). St Louis: Mosby.

Burgess, A. (1997) *Fatherhood Reclaimed: The Making of the Modern Father*. London: Vermilion.

Burghes, L., Clarke, L. and Cronin, N. (1997) *Fathers and Fatherhood in Britain*. London: Family Policy Studies Centre.

Cahill, H. (2001) Male appropriation and medicalisation of childbirth: an historical analysis. *Journal of Advanced Nursing* 33 (3): 334–42.

Campbell, J. and Johnston, C. (1999) Trend spotting: fashions in medical education. *British Medical Journal* 318 (7193): 1272–5.

Campbell, R. (1997) Place of birth reconsidered (ch. 1), in J. Alexander, V. Levy and C. Roth (eds) *Midwifery Practice. Core Topics 2*. London: Macmillan.

Campbell, R. and MacFarlane, A. (1987) *Where to be born? – The Debate and the Evidence*. Oxford: National Perinatal Epidemiology Unit.

Campbell, S. and Little, D.J. (1980) Clinical potential of real-time ultrasound (ch. 5), in M.J. Bennett and S. Campbell (eds) *Real-Time Ultrasound in Obstetrics*. Oxford: Blackwell Scientific Publications.

Capstick, B. and Edwards, P. (1991) Defensive obstetric practice. *Lancet* 338 (8770): 823.

Carter, J. and Duriez, T. (1986) *With Child: Birth Through the Ages*. Edinburgh: Mainstream.

Catanzariti, R. (2001) Can you refuse to employ a male midwife? Reprinted from the VHA Report with permission of the Victorian Healthcare Association and Phillips Fox Lawyers. *Australian Midwifery News* 1 (1): 5.

CEMD (1998) *Why Mothers Die: The Confidential Enquiries into Maternal Deaths in the United Kingdom 1994–1996*. Royal College of Obstetricians and Gynaecologists.

CEMD (2001) *Why Mothers Die 1999–1997: The Confidential Enquiries into Maternal Deaths in the United Kingdom*. Royal College of Obstetricians and Gynaecologists.

Chapman, L.L. (1992) Expectant fathers' roles during labor and birth. *Journal of Obstetric Gynecological and Neonatal Nursing* 21 (2): 114–20.

Chodorow, N. (1978) *The Reproduction of Mothering: Psychoanalysis and the Sociology of Gender*. Berkeley: University of California Press.

Cochrane, A.L. (1972) *Effectiveness and Efficiency*. London: Nuffield Provincial Hospitals Trust.

Cogan, R., Henneborn, W. and Klopfer, F. (1976) Predictors of pain during prepared childbirth. *Journal of Psychosomatic Research* 20 (6): 523–33.

Corea, G. (1977) *The Hidden Malpractice: How American Medicine Mistreats Women*. New York: Jove/HBI.

Correspondence (1977) Husband at the delivery. *Midwives Chronicle* January: 9–11.

Courtenay, W.H. (2000) Constructions of masculinity and their influence on men's well-being: a theory of gender and health. *Social Science and Medicine* 50: 1385–401.

Cronenwett, L.R. and Newmark, L.L. (1974) Fathers' responses to childbirth. *Nursing Research* 23(3): 210–17.

Cruz, J.M. and Firestone, J.M. (1998) Exploring violence and abuse in gay male relationships. *Violence and Victims* 13 (2): 159–73.

Cunningham, A. (2002) Thoemmes Press: the history of ideas. http://www.thoemmes. com/encyclopedia/harvey.htm. Accessed 6 February.

Daly, K.J. (1995) Reshaping fatherhood: finding the models (ch. 2, p. 21), in W. Marsiglio (ed.) *Fatherhood: Contemporary Theory, Research and Social Policy.* Thousand Oaks, CA: Sage.

Davis-Floyd, R. and Sargent, C. (1997) *Childbirth and Authoritative Knowledge: Cross-Cultural Perspectives.* Berkeley: University of California Press.

Deane-Gray, T. (2001) A phenomenological examination of the experience of fathers-to-be in labour. Unpublished MA dissertation, City University.

DeLee, J.B. (1920) The prophylactic forceps operation. *American Journal of Obstetrics and Gynaecology* 1: 34–44.

DeVries, R. (1996) The midwife's place: an international comparison of the status of midwives (ch. 13, p. 159), in S. Murray (ed.) *Midwives and Safer Motherhood.* St Louis: Mosby.

DHSS (1970) *Domiciliary Midwifery and Maternity Bed Needs: the Report of the Standing Maternity and Midwifery Advisory Committee* (Subcommittee Chairman J. Peel). London: Department of Health and Social Security, HMSO.

Dick-Reed, G. (1942) *Natural Childbirth.* London: Heinemann.

Diemer, G.A. (1997) Expectant fathers: influence of perinatal education on stress, coping and spousal relations. *Research in Nursing and Health* 20 (4): 281–93.

Dixon, M. (1977) Letter: Husband at the delivery. *Midwives Chronicle* November: 269.

Dixon, R. (2000) Midwives as 'mid-husbands'? Midwives and fathers (ch. 12, pp. 270–87), in J. Bornat, R. Perks, P. Thompson and J. Walmsley (eds) *Oral History, Health and Welfare.* London and New York: Routledge.

Dobash, R.E., Dobash, R.P., Cavanagh, K. and Lewis, R. (2000) *Changing Violent Men.* Thousand Oaks, CA: Sage.

DoH (1998) *A First Class Service.* Leeds: Department of Health, NHS Executive.

DoH (1999) Confidential enquiries into maternal deaths. http://www.doh.gov.uk/ cmo/mdeaths.htm#introduction. Accessed 15 August 2002.

Donnison, J. (1973) *Midwives and Medical Men – A History of Interprofessional Rivalry and Women's Rights.* London: Heinemann.

Donnison, J. (1988) *Midwives and Medical Men: A History of the Struggle for the Control of Childbirth* (2nd edn). New Barnet: Historical Publications.

Douglas, M. (1966) *Purity and Danger: An Analysis of the Concepts of Pollution and Taboo.* London: Routledge & Kegan Paul.

Draper, J. (1997) Whose welfare in the labour room? A discussion of the increasing trend of fathers' birth attendance. *Midwifery* 13 (3): 132–8.

Draper, J. (2002) 'It's the first scientific evidence': men's experience of pregnancy confirmation. *Journal of Advanced Nursing* 39 (6): 563–70.

Dunn, P.M. (1999) The Chamberlen family (1560–1728) and obstetric forceps. *Archives of Disease in Childhood* (Foetal Neonatal edn) 81: F232–5.

Dyregrov, A. (1991) *Grief in Children: A Handbook for Adults*. London: Jessica Kingsley.

Earle, S. (2000) Why some women do not breast feed: bottle feeding and fathers' role. *Midwifery* 16 (4): 323–30.

Edin, K.E. and Högberg, U. (2002) Violence against pregnant women will remain hidden as long as no direct questions are asked. *Midwifery* 18 (4): 268–78.

Edinburgh University (2002) University of Edinburgh, Secretary's Office – Planning Section website: http://www.planning.ed.ac.uk/Profile/200102/genderchart.htm. Accessed 15 February.

English National Board (2001) Placements in focus: developments in multiprofessional education (ENB and DoH). http://www.doh.gov.uk/pdfs/places.pdf. Accessed 8 July 2003.

Entwistle, D.R. and Doering, S.G. (1981) *The First Birth*. Baltimore, MD: Johns Hopkins University Press.

Erikson, E. (1963) *Childhood and Society*. Toronto: Norton.

Erikson, E (1982) *Identity and the Life Cycle*. New York: Norton.

Etzion, D. (1984) Moderating effect of social support on the stress burnout relationship. *Journal of Applied Psychology* 69 (4): 615–22.

Fathers Direct (2002) http://www.europrofem.org/02.info/22contri/2.04.en/2en.masc/33en_mas.htm. Accessed 14 July 2003.

Fawdry, R. (1994) Midwives and the care of 'normal' childbirth. *British Journal of Midwifery* 2 (7): 302–3.

Finch, J. (2000) Interprofessional education and teamworking: a view from the education providers. *British Medical Journal* 321: 1138–40.

Fleming, V. (2002) Statutory control (ch. 4, pp. 63–77) in R. Mander and V. Fleming (eds) *Failure to Progress: The Contraction of the Midwifery Profession*. London: Routledge.

Flynn, J. (1977) Recent findings related to wife abuse. *Social Case Work* 63: 40–7.

Foucault, M. (1963) *Birth of the Clinic*. London: Tavistock.

Foy, R., Nelson, F., Penney, G. and McIlwaine, G. (2000) Antenatal detection of domestic violence (Letter). *Lancet* 355: 1915.

Frank, D.I. (1984) Counselling the infertile couple. *Journal of Psychosocial Nursing* 22 (5): 17–23.

Fraser, W.D., Turcot, L., Krauss, I. and Brisson-Carrol, G. (2002) Amniotomy for shortening spontaneous labour (Cochrane Review), in *The Cochrane Library*, Issue 4. Chichester: John Wiley & Sons.

Frazer, J.G. (1922) *The Golden Bough: A Study in Magic and Religion*. London: Macmillan.

Freed, G.L., Fraley, J.K. and Schanler, R.J. (1992) Attitudes of expectant fathers regarding breast-feeding. *Pediatrics* 90 (2): 224–7.

French, S. (1995) The fallen idol (ch. 1, pp. 1–8), in P. Moss (ed.) *Father Figures: Fathers in the Families of the 1990s*. Edinburgh: HMSO.

Gamble, D. and Morse, J.M. (1993) Fathers of breastfed infants: postponing and types of involvement. *Journal of Obstetric, Gynecological and Neonatal Nursing* 22 (4): 358–65.

Garcia, J. and Garforth, S. (1989) Labour and delivery routines in English consultant maternity units. *Midwifery* 5 (4): 155–62.

Garcia, J. and Davidson, L. (2002) Researching domestic violence and health: National Perinatal Epidemiology unit. *MIDIRS Midwifery Digest* 12 (Supp 2): S25–S29.

Gielen A.C., O'Campo, P.J., Faden, R.R., Kass, N.E. and Xue, X. (1994) Interpersonal conflict and physical violence during the childbearing year. *Social Science and Medicine* 39 (6): 781–7.

Gillis, J.R. (1997) *A World of Their Own Making: A History of Myth and Ritual in Family Life*. Oxford: Oxford University Press.

Gillis, J.R. (2000) Marginalisation of fatherhood in western countries. *Childhood* 7 (2): 225–38.

Glover, L., Abel, P.D., and Gannon, K. (1998) Male subfertility: is pregnancy the only issue? *British Medical Journal* 316: 1405–6.

Glover, L., Gannon, K. and Abel, P.D. (1999) Eighteen month follow up of male subfertility clinic attenders: a comparison between men whose partners subsequently became pregnant and those with continuing subfertility. *Journal of Reproductive and Infant Psychology* 17 (1): 83–7.

Glover, L., Gannon, K., Sherr, L. and Abel, P.D. (1996) Distress in sub-fertile men: a longitudinal study. *Journal of Reproductive and Infant Psychology* 14 (1): 23–36.

Goer, H. (1995) *Obstetric Myths Versus Research Realities*. Westport, CT: Bergin & Garvey.

Goleman, D. (1996) *Emotional Intelligence: Why It Can Matter More than IQ*. London: Bloomsbury Publishing.

Gough, B. (2001) 'Biting your tongue': negotiating masculinities in contemporary Britain. *Journal of Gender Studies* 10 (2): 169–85.

Gould, D. (2000) Normal labour: a concept analysis. *Journal of Advanced Nursing* 31 (2): 418–27.

Graham, H. (1969) *Eternal Eve*. London: Hutchinson.

Graham, I.D. (1997) *Episiotomy: Challenging Obstetric Interventions*. Oxford: Blackwell Science.

Green, J., Statham, H. and Snowdon, C. (1992) Screening for fetal abnormalities: attitudes and experiences (ch. 5, p. 65), in T. Chard and M.P.M. Richards (eds) *Obstetrics in the 1990s: Current controversies*. Oxford: Mackeith Press and Blackwell Scientific.

Greenhalgh, R., Slade, P. and Spiby, H. (2000) Fathers' coping style, antenatal preparation and experiences of labour and the puerperium. *Birth* 27 (3): 177–84.

Greil, A.L. (1997) Infertility and psychological distress: a critical review of the literature. *Social Science and Medicine* 45 (11): 1679–704.

Halford, S., Savage, M. and With, A. (1997) *Gender, Careers and Organisations: Current Development in Banking, Nursing and Local Government*. Basingstoke: Macmillan.

Hall, J. (1993) Attendance not compulsory. *Nursing Times* 89 (46): 69–71.

Hallgren, A., Kihlgren, M., Forslin, L. and Norberg, A. (1999) Swedish fathers' involvement in and experiences of childbirth preparation and childbirth. *Midwifery* 15 (1): 6–15.

Harcombe, J. (1999) Power and political power positions in maternity care. *British Journal of Midwifery* 7 (2): 78–81.

Harris, K. (1984) *Sex, Ideology and Religion: The Representation of Women in the Bible*. New Jersey: Barnes & Noble.

Harris, R. (1994) The process of infertility (ch. 2, pp. 15–81), in P.A. Field and P.B. Marck (eds) *Uncertain Motherhood: Negotiating the Risks of the Childbearing Years*. Thousand Oaks, CA: Sage.

Harrison, S., Hunter, D.J., Marnoch, G. and Pollitt, C. (1992) *Just Managing: Power and Culture in the National Health Service*. London: Macmillan.

Hawkins, A.J., Christiansen, S.L., Sargent, K.P. and Hill, E.J. (1995) Rethinking fathers' involvement in child care: a developmental perspective (ch. 3, p. 41) in W. Marsiglio (ed.) *Fatherhood: Contemporary Theory Research and Social Policy*. Thousand Oaks, CA: Sage.

Hawkins J.W. and Higgins L.P. (1981) *Maternity and Gynecological Nursing: Women's Health Care*. Philadelphia, PA: Lippincott.

Helton, A.S. and Snodgrass, F.G. (1987) Battering during pregnancy: intervention strategies. *Birth* 14 (3): 142–7.

Hewson, B. (1994) Court-ordered caesarean: ethical triumph or surgical rape? *AIMS Journal* 6 (2): 1–5.

Hicks, C. (1992) Research in midwifery: are midwives their own worst enemies? *Midwifery* 8 (1): 12–18.

Hill, M. (1987) *Sharing Child Care in Early Parenthood*. London: Routledge & Kegan Paul.

Hondagneu-Sotelo, P. and Messner, M.A. (1994) Gender displays and men's power (ch. 11, p. 200), in H. Brod and M. Kaufman (eds) *Theorizing Masculinities*. London: Sage.

Howarth, G. R. and Botha, D. J. (2002) Amniotomy plus intravenous oxytocin for induction of labour (Cochrane Review), in *The Cochrane Library*, Issue 4. Chichester: John Wiley & Sons.

Howe, A., Billingham, K. and Walters, C. (2002) In our own image – a multi-disciplinary qualitative analysis of medical education. *Journal of Interprofessional Care* 16 (4): 379–89.

Howell, C.J. and Chalmers, I. (1992) A review of prospectively controlled comparisons of epidural with non-epidural forms of pain relief during labour. *International Journal of Obstetrical Anaesthesia* 1: 93–110.

Illich, I. (1997) *Limits to Medicine*. Harmondsworth: Penguin.

Ip, Wy (2000) Relationships between partner's support during labour and maternal outcomes. *Journal of Clinical Nursing* 9 (2): 265–72.

IPPF (2002) *Safe Motherhood* (ch. 3): http://www.ippf.org/resource/refugeehealth/manual/3a2.htm. Accessed 20 February.

Isherwood, K. (2000/1) Home birth is not an 'optional extra'. *AIMS Journal* 12 (4): 22.

Jackson, B. (1984) *Fatherhood*. London: George Allen & Unwin.

Jackson, C. and Mander, R. (1995) History or herstory: the decline and fall of the midwife? *British Journal of Midwifery* 3 (5): 279–83.

Jackson, K.B. (1997) Men and midwifery. Paternal presence at delivery. *British Journal of Midwifery* 5 (11): 682–4.

Jacobs, K. (2003) Personal communication.

Jeffery, P. and Jeffery, R. (1996) Delayed periods and falling babies (ch. 1, pp. 17–38), in R. Cecil (ed.) *The Anthropology of Pregnancy Loss*. Oxford: Berg.

Jeffery, P., Jeffery, R. and Lyon, A. (1989) *Labour Pains and Labour Power*. London: Zed Books.

Johnson, M.P. (2002a) The implications of unfulfilled expectations and perceived pressure to attend the birth on men's stress levels following birth attendance: a longitudinal study. *Journal of Psychosomatic Obstetrics and Gynecology* 23 (3): 173–82.

Johnson, M.P. (2002b) An exploration of men's experience and role at childbirth. *Journal of Men's Studies* 10 (2): 165–82.

Jonquil, S.G. (1993) Preparing siblings. *Midwifery Today and Childbirth Education* 28 (Winter): 34–5.

Jordan, B. (1997) Authoritative knowledge and its construction (ch. 1), in R.E. Davis-Floyd and C.F. Sargent (eds) *Childbirth and Authoritative Knowledge: Cross-Cultural Perspectives* Berkeley: University of California Press.

Jordan, P.L. and Wall, V.R. (1990) Breast feeding and fathers: illuminating the darker side. *Birth* 17 (4): 210–17.

Kargar, I. (1990) Traditional midwifery skills. *Nursing Times* 86 (23), Supplement, *Midwives' Journal*: 74–5.

Keele, K.D. (1965) *William Harvey: The Man, The Physician and the Scientist*. London: Nelson.

Keirse, M.J.N.C. (1986) Electronic monitoring in labour: too good to be put to the test? *Birth* 13 (4): 256–8.

King, H. (1983) Bound to bleed: Artemis and Greek women (ch. 8, pp. 109–27), in A. Cameron and A. Kuhrt (eds) *Images of Women in Antiquity*. London: Croom Helm.

Kirkham, M. (1986) A feminist perspective in midwifery (ch. 3, pp. 35–49), in C. Webb (ed.) *Feminist Practice in Women's Health Care*. Chichester: John Wiley.

Kitzinger, J.V. (1992) Counteracting, not re-enacting, the violation of women's bodies: the challenge for perinatal caregivers. *Birth* 19 (4): 219–20.

Kitzinger, J.V., Green, J.M. and Coupland, V.A. (1993) Labour relations: midwives and doctors on the labour ward (ch. 6), in J. Walmsley, J. Reynolds, P. Shakespeare and R. Woolfe (eds) *Health Welfare and Practice: Reflecting on Roles and Relationships*. London: Sage.

Kitzinger, S. (1972) *The Experience of Childbirth*. London: Victor Gollancz.

Kitzinger, S (1989) Perceptions of pain in home and hospital birth (pp. 90–100), in E.V. van Hall and W. Everaerd (eds) *The Free Woman: Women's Health in the 1990s*. Parthenon: Carnforth.

Kitzinger, S. (1992) Birth and violence against women (ch.4, pp. 63–80), in H. Roberts (ed.) *Women's Health Matters*. London: Routledge.

Kitzinger, S. (1994) *Ourselves as Mothers*. Boston, MA: Addison-Wesley.

Kitzinger, S. (2000) Some cultural perspectives of birth. *British Journal of Midwifery* 8 (12): 746–50.

Klein, H. (1991) Couvade syndrome – Male counterpart to pregnancy. *International Journal of Psychiatry in Medicine* 21 (1): 57–69.

Koppel, G.T. and Kaiser, D. (2001) Fathers at the end of their rope: a brief report of fathers abandoned in the perinatal situation. *Journal of Reproductive and Infant Psychology* 19 (3): 249–51.

Kurz, T. (1997) Doing parenting: Mothers care work and policy (ch. 4, p. 92), in

T. Arendell (ed.) *Contemporary Parenting: Challenges and Issues*. Thousand Oaks, CA: Sage.

Laderman, C. (1988) Commentary: cross-cultural perspectives on birth practice. *Birth* 15 (2): 86–7.

Lamb, M.E. (1986) The changing role of fathers (ch. 1, pp. 3–27), in M.E. Lamb (ed.) *The Father's Role: Applied Perspectives*. New York: Wiley.

Larossa, R. (1997) *The Modernization of Fatherhood: A Social and Political History*. Chicago, IL: University of Chicago Press.

Lavender, T., Wallymahmed, A.H. and Walkinshaw, S.A. (1999) Managing labour using partograms with different action lines: a prospective study of women's views. *Birth* 26 (2): 89–98.

Leap, N. and Hunter, B. (1993) *The Midwife's Tale: An Oral History from Handywoman to Professional Midwife*. London: Scarlet Press.

Leaviss, J. (2000) Exploring the perceived effect of an undergraduate multiprofessional educational intervention. *Medical Education* 34 (6): 483–6.

Lee T.-Y. and Chu, T-Y (2001) The Chinese experience of male infertility. *Western Journal of Nursing Research* 23 (7): 714–25.

Lee T-Y., Sun, G-H and Chao, S-C. (2001) The effect of an infertility diagnosis on the distress, marital and sexual satisfaction between husbands and wives in Taiwan. *Human Reproduction* 16 (8): 1762–7.

Lester, A. and Moorsom, S. (1997) Men and midwifery. Do men need midwives: facilitating a greater involvement in parenting. *British Journal of Midwifery* 5 (11): 678–81.

Lewis, C. (1996) *Becoming a Father*. Milton Keynes: Open University Press.

Lewis, G. (2001) Domestic violence (ch. 16, p. 241), in RCOG (eds) *Why Mothers Die 1997–1999: The Confidential Enquiries into Maternal Deaths in the United Kingdom*. Royal College of Obstetricians and Gynaecologists.

Lewis, P. (1989) Male midwives: reasons for training and subsequent career paths (ch. 28, pp. 280–9), in J. Wilson-Barnett and S. Robinson (eds) *Directions in Nursing Research*. London: Scutari Press.

Lewis, P. (1991) Men in midwifery: their experiences as students and as practitioners (ch. 10, p. 271) in S. Robinson and A.M. Thomson (eds) *Midwives, Research and Childbirth*, Vol. 2. London: Chapman and Hall.

Lewis, P. (1998) What makes a man become a midwife?, in M. Robotham, Delivery men. *Nursing Times* 94 (17): 62–4.

Littman, H., Medendorp, S. and Goldfarb, J. (1994) The decision to breastfeed: the importance of a father's approval. *Clinical Pediatrics* 33 (4): 214–19.

Lloyd, S. (1997) Defining violence against women (ch. 1), in S. Bewley, J. Friend and G. Mezey (eds) *Violence Against Women*. London: RCOG Press.

Lloyd, T. (1995) Fathers in the media: an analysis of newspaper coverage of fathers (ch. 5, p. 41), in P. Moss (ed.) *Father Figures: Fathers in the Families of the 1990s*. Edinburgh: HMSO.

Lorber, J. (1993) Why women physicians will never be true equals in the American medical profession (ch. 3, pp. 62–76), in E. Riska, and K. Wegar (eds) *Gender, Work and Medicine: Women and the Medical Division of Labour*. London: Sage.

Lorber, J. (1997) *Gender and the Social Construction of Illness*. Thousand Oaks, CA: Sage.

Loudon, I. (1992) *Death in Childbirth*. Oxford: Clarendon Press.

Lummis, T. (1982) The historical dimension of fatherhood: a case study 1890–1914 (ch. 3), in L. McKee and M. O'Brien (eds) *The Father Figure*. London: Tavistock.

Lunn, S. (2002) Wet nursing – the story of two mums and a baby. *ABM Natural Parent* online magazine http://home.clara.net/abm/pages/magazine/wetnurse.htm. Accessed 18 July.

Lupton, D. and Barclay, L. (1997) *Constructing Fatherhood: Discourses and Experiences*. London: Sage.

McClain, C. (1982) Toward a comparative framework for the study of childbirth: a review of the literature (ch. 2, p. 25), in M.A. Kay (ed.) *Anthropology of Human Birth*. Philadelphia, PA: F.A. Davis.

McClellan, A.C. and Killeen, M.R. (2000) Attachment theory and violence toward women by male intimate partners *Journal of Nursing Scholarship* (Fourth Quarter): 353–60.

McCracken, B. (1999) A father's anger and birth love. http://www.compleatmother. com/father's_anger.htm. Accessed 22 May 2002.

MacDonald, A.M. (1981) *Chambers Twentieth Century Dictionary*. Edinburgh: Chambers.

MacFarlane, A. (1977) *The Psychology of Childbirth*. London: Fontana.

McFarlane, J., Parker, B., Soeken, K. and Bullock, L. (1992) Assessing for abuse during pregnancy. *Journal of the American Medical Association* 267 (23): 3176.

McFarlane, J., Soeken, K. and Wiist, W. (2000) An evaluation of interventions to decrease intimate partner violence to pregnant women. *Public Health Nursing* 17 (6): 443–51.

MacInnes, J. (1998) *The End of Masculinity: The Confusion of Sexual Genesis and Sexual Difference in Modern Society*. Buckingham: Open University Press.

McKee, L. and O'Brien, M. (1982) The father figure: some current orientations and historical perspectives (ch. 1), in L. McKee and M. O'Brien (eds) *The Father Figure*. London: Tavistock.

MacMillan, M. (1994) *Men at Birth*. London: Royal College of Midwives Survey.

McWilliams, M. and McKiernan, J. (1993) *Bringing it Out Into the Open: Domestic Violence in Northern Ireland*. Belfast: HMSO.

Mander, G. (2001) Fatherhood today: variations on a theme. *Psychodynamic Counselling* 7 (2): 141–58.

Mander, R. (1988) What can midwives learn from the babes? Implications for midwives of a maternity care programme for nursing students. *Journal of Advanced Nursing* 13 (3): 306–13.

Mander, R. (1989) A maternity care course component and evaluation. *Nurse Education Today* 9 (4): 227–35.

Mander, R. (1993) Epidural analgesia 1. Recent history. *British Journal of Midwifery* 1 (6): 259–64.

Mander, R. (1994a) Epidural analgesia 2. Research basis. *British Journal of Midwifery* 2 (1): 12–16.

Mander, R. (1994b) *Loss and Bereavement in Childbearing*. Oxford: Blackwell Scientific.

Mander, R. (1995) *The Care of the Mother Grieving a Baby Relinquished for Adoption*. Aldershot: Avebury.

Mander, R. (2001a) *Supportive Care and Midwifery*. Oxford: Blackwell Science.

Mander, R. (2001b) The midwife's ultimate paradox: a UK-based study of the death of a mother. *Midwifery* 17 (4): 248–59.

Mander, R. and Reid, L. (2002) Midwifery power (ch. 1, pp. 1–19), in R. Mander and V. Fleming (eds) *Failure to Progress: The Contraction of the Midwifery Profession*. London: Routledge.

Marck, P.B. (1994) Unexpected pregnancy: the uncharted land of women's experience (ch. 3, pp. 82–138) in P.A. Field and P.B. Marck (eds) *Uncertain Motherhood: Negotiating the Risks of the Childbearing Years*. Thousand Oaks, CA: Sage.

Marsiglio, W. (1995) Fatherhood scholarship: an overview and agenda for the future (ch. 1, p. 1) in W. Marsiglio (ed.) *Fatherhood: Contemporary Theory, Research and Social Policy*. Thousand Oaks, CA: Sage.

Martin, E. (1987) *The Woman in the Body*. Milton Keynes: Open University Press.

Mason, C. and Elwood, R. (1995) Is there a physiological basis for the couvade and onset of paternal care? *International Journal of Nursing Studies* 32 (2): 137–48.

Mason, J. (2000) Letter: Midwives 'verging on the sadistic'. *British Journal of Midwifery* 8 (4): 247.

May, K. (1982) Three phases of father involvement. *Pregnancy Nursing Research* 30 (6): 337.

Mead, M. and Newton, N. (1967) Cultural patterning of parental behaviour (pp. 142–245), in S.A. Richardson and A.F. Guttmacher (eds) *Childbearing – Its Social and Psychological Aspects*. Baltimore, MD: Williams & Wilkins.

Melzack, R. (1993) Pain: past, present and future. *Canadian Journal of Experimental Psychology* 47 (4): 615–29.

Menning, B.E. (1982) The psychosocial impact of infertility. *The Nursing Clinics of North America* 17 (1): 155–63.

Mezey, G.C. (1997a) Perpetrators of domestic violence (ch. 4, p. 35) in S. Bewley, J. Friend and G. Mezey (eds) *Violence Against Women*. London: RCOG Press.

Mezey, G.C. (1997b) Domestic violence in pregnancy (ch. 21, p. 191), in S. Bewley, J. Friend and G. Mezey (eds) *Violence Against Women*. London: RCOG Press.

Mezey, G.C. and Bewley, S. (2000) An exploration of the prevalence and effects of domestic violence in pregnancy (ESRC). http://www.regard.ac.uk/research_findings/L133251043/report.pdf Accessed 16 August 2002.

Middleton, K. (2000) How Karembola men become mothers (ch. 6, pp. 104–27), in J. Carsten (ed.) *Cultures of Relatedness: New Approaches to the Study of Kinship*. Cambridge: Cambridge University Press.

Migliaccio, T.A. (2002) Abused husbands – a narrative analysis. *Journal of Family Issues* 23 (1): 26–52.

Millett, K. (1971) *Sexual Politics*. London: Rupert Hart-Davis.

Mold J.W. and Stein, H.F. (1986) The cascade effect in the clinical care of patients. *New England Journal of Medicine* 314 (8): 512–14.

Mooney, J. (1995) The method used and a selection of the findings from the North London Domestic Violence Survey. Occasional Paper. *Centre for Criminology*, Middlesex University.

Mooney, J. (2000) *Gender, Violence and the Social Order*. Basingstoke, Macmillan.

Moore, W. (2000) Birthday boys. *Observer*, 9 July. http://www.observer.co.uk/Print/0,3858,4038418,00.html. Accessed 8 February 2002.

Moss, P. (1995) *Father Figures: Fathers in the Families of the 1990s*. Edinburgh: HMSO.

Murphy, F.A. (1998) The experience of early miscarriage from a male perspective. *Journal of Clinical Nursing* 7 (4): 325–32.

Murphy-Black, T. (1990) Introduction (ch. 1), in A. Faulkner and T. Murphy-Black (eds) *Midwifery: Excellence in Nursing – the Research Route*. London: Scutari.

National Childbirth Trust (1998) Your role at the birth. http://www.nctpregnancy andbabycare.com/article.asp?article=98. Accessed 11 July 2003.

Neilson, J.P. (2002) Ultrasound for fetal assessment in early pregnancy (Cochrane Review), in *The Cochrane Library*, Issue 1. Oxford: Update Software.

Nichols, M.R. (1993) Paternal perspectives of the childbirth experience. *Maternal-Child Nursing Journal* 21 (3): 99–108.

Niven, C. (1985) How helpful is the presence of the husband at the birth. *Journal of Reproduction and Infant Psychology* 3: 45–53.

Niven, C.A. (1992) *Psychological Care for Families: Before, During and After Birth*. Oxford: Butterworth Heinemann.

Nolan, M. (1994) Caring for fathers in antenatal classes. *Modern Midwife* 4 (2): 25–8.

Nolan, M. (1998) *Antenatal Education: a Dynamic Approach* (ch. 9). London: Baillière Tindall.

Norton, L.B., Peipert, J.F., Zierler, S., Lima, B. and Hume, L. (1995) Battering in pregnancy: an assessment of two screening methods. *Obstetrics and Gynecology* 85 (3): 321–5.

O'Driscoll, K. and Meagher, D. (1986) *Active Management of Labour* (2nd edn). London: Baillière Tindall.

O'Driscoll, K., Meagher, D. and Boylan, P. (1993) Active Management of Labour: The Dublin Experience (3rd edn). London: Mosby.

Oakley, A. (1982) The origins and development of antenatal care (ch. 1), in M. Enkin and I. Chalmers (eds) *Effectiveness and Satisfaction in Antenatal Care*. London: SIMP.

Oakley, A. (1984) *The Captured Womb: A History of the Medical Care of Pregnant Women*. Oxford: Blackwell.

Oakley, A. (1989) Who cares for women? Science versus love in midwifery today. *Midwives Chronicle* 102 (1218): 214–21.

Oakley, A. (1993) Ways of knowing: feminism and the challenge to knowledge (ch. 16, p. 203), in A. Oakley *Essays on Women, Medicine and Health*. Edinburgh: Edinburgh University Press.

Oakley, A. and Richards, M.P.M. (1990) Caesarean deliveries (ch. 10), in J. Garcia, R. Kilpatrick and M. Richards (eds) *The Politics of Maternity Care*. Oxford: Clarendon Press.

Oakley, A., McPherson, A. and Roberts, H. (1990) *Miscarriage*. London: Penguin.

O'Bryant, C. (2001) Portrait of a male midwife. *Midwifery Today* 58: 33.

Odent, M. (1987) The fetus ejection reflex. *Birth* 14 (2): 104–5.

Odent, M. (1999) Is the participation of the father at the birth dangerous? *Midwifery Today* 51: 23–4.

Olsen, O. and Jewell, M.D. (2002) Home versus hospital birth (Cochrane Review), in *The Cochrane Library*, Issue 1. Oxford: Update Software.

Palkowitz, R. Copes, M.A. and Woolfolk, T.N. (2001) Men and Masculinities 4 (1): 49–69.

Perkins, E.R. (1980) *Men on the Labour Ward*. University of Nottingham: Leverhulme.

Philpott, R.H. (1972) Graphic records in labour. *British Medical Journal* 4: 163–5.

Pitt, S. (1997) Midwifery and Medicine: Gendered knowledge in the practice of delivery (ch. 10, pp. 218–31) in H. Marland and A.M. Rafferty (eds) *Midwives, Society and Childbirth*. London: Routledge.

Pizzey, E. (1974) *Scream Quietly or the Neighbours Will Hear*, edited by Alison Forbes. Harmondsworth: Penguin.

Podkolinski, J. (1998) Women's experience of postnatal support (ch. 11, p. 205), in S. Clement (ed.) *Psychological Perspectives on Pregnancy and Childbirth*. Edinburgh: Churchill Livingstone.

Pollack, S. and Sutton, J. (1985) Fathers' rights, women's losses. *Women's Studies International Forum* 8 (6): 593–9.

Prendiville, W.J., Elbourne, D. and McDonald, S. (2002) Active versus expectant management in the third stage of labour (Cochrane Review), in *The Cochrane Library*, Issue 1. Oxford: Update Software.

Price, S. and Baird, K. (2001) Domestic violence in pregnancy: how can midwives make a difference. *Practising Midwife* 4 (7): 12–14.

Puddifoot, J.E. and Johnson, M.P. (1997) The legitimacy of grieving: the partner's experience at miscarriage. *Social Science and Medicine* 45 (6): 837–45.

Puddifoot, J.E. and Johnson, M.P. (1999) Active grief, despair, and difficulty coping: Some measured characteristics of male response following their partner's miscarriage. *Journal of Reproductive and Infant Psychology* 17 (2): 89–94.

Ramsay, J., Richardson, J., Carter, Y.H., Davidson, L.L. and Feder, G. (2002) Should health professionals screen women for domestic violence? Systematic review. *British Medical Journal* 325: 314–27.

Ranson, G. (2001) Men at work: change – or no change? – in the era of the 'New Father'. *Men and Masculinities* 4 (1): 3–26.

RCM (1995a) RCM survey – 'Men at birth'. *Midwives* 108 (1284): 18.

RCM (1995b) *Select Reading List: Fathers and Siblings at the Birth*. London: Royal College of Midwives.

RCM (1998) *Domestic Abuse in Pregnancy Position*. Paper No. 19. London: Royal College of Midwives.

RCOG (2002) Brief history of the College. http://www.rcog.org.uk/history.html. Accessed 26 February.

Reeves, H. and Baden, S. (2000) Gender and development: concepts and definitions. Bridge development – gender. University of Sussex. http://www.ids.ac.uk/bridge/reports_gend_con_meth.htm. Accessed 10 July 2003.

Reeves, S., Freeth, D., McCrorie, P. and Perry, D. (2002) 'It teaches you what to expect in future . . .': interprofessional learning on a training ward for medical, nursing, occupational therapy and physiotherapy students. *Medical Education* 36 (4): 337–44.

Reid, M. (1990) Prenatal diagnosis and screening: a review (ch. 16, p. 300), in J. Garcia, R. Kilpatrick and M. Richards (eds) *The Politics of Maternity Care Services for Childbearing Women in Twentieth Century Britain*. Oxford: Clarendon Press.

Richman, J. (1982) Men's experiences of pregnancy and childbirth (ch. 6, pp. 89–103), in L. McKee and M. O'Brien (eds) *The Father Figure*. London: Tavistock.

Robertson, A. (1999) Get the fathers involved! The needs of men in pregnancy classes. *Practising Midwife* 2 (1): 21–2.

Robotham, M. (1998) Delivery men. *Nursing Times* 94 (17): 62–4.

Rosser, J. (1994) World Health Organisation Partograph in management of labour. *MIDIRS Midwifery Digest* 4 (4): 436–7.

Rozario, S. (1992) *Purity and Communal Boundaries: Women and Social Change in a Bangladeshi Village.* London: Zed Books.

Samuelsson, M., Radestad, I. and Segesten, K. (2001) A waste of life: Fathers' experience of losing a child before birth. *Birth* 28 (2): 124–30.

Sanz, J. (2001) Spain: the story of a male midwife. *Midwifery Today* 57: 57.

Sargent, L. (2002) Practice and autonomy (ch. 3, pp. 39–62), in R. Mander and V. Fleming (eds) *Failure to Progress: The Contraction of the Midwifery Profession.* London: Routledge.

Savage, W. (1998) The right to choose. *Nursing Standard* 12 (35): 14.

Scobie, J. and McGuire, M. (1999) The silent enemy: domestic violence in pregnancy. *British Journal of Midwifery* 7 (4): 259–62.

Scott, J.A., Binns, C.W. and Aron, R.A. (1997) The influence of reported paternal attitudes on the decision to breast-feed. *Journal of Paediatrics and Child Health* 33 (3): 305–7.

Scott-Heyes, G. (1983) Marital adaptation during pregnancy and after childbirth. *Journal of Reproductive and Infant Psychology* 1 (1): 18–28.

Scully, D. (1994) *Men Who Control Women's Health: The Miseducation of Obstetrician-Gynecologists.* New York: Athene.

Segal, L. (1990) *Slow Motion: Changing Masculinities, Changing Men.* New Brunswick, NJ: Rutgers University Press.

Seidler, V.J. (1997) *Man Enough: Embodying Masculinities.* London: Sage.

Shapiro, M.C., Nazman, J.M., Chang, A., Keeping, J.D., Morrison, J. and Western, J.S. (1983) Information control and the exercise of power in the obstetrical encounter. *Social Science and Medicine* 17 (3): 139–46.

Sheahan, D. (1972) The game of the name. *Nursing Outlook* 20 (7): 440–4.

Shorter, E. (1983) *A History of Women's Bodies.* London: Allen Lane.

Simkin, P. (1986) Is anyone listening? The lack of clinical impact of randomized controlled trials of electronic fetal monitoring. *Birth* 13 (4): 219–20.

Singh, D. and Newburn, M. (2000) Becoming a father: men's access to information and support about pregnancy birth and life with a new baby. National Childbirth Trust with Fathers Direct.

Smith, J. (1995) The first intruder: fatherhood a historical perspective (ch. 3, p. 17), in P. Moss (ed.) *Father Figures: Fathers in Families of the 1990s.* Edinburgh: HMSO.

Smith, J. (1999b) Antenatal classes and the transition to fatherhood: a study of some fathers' views. *MIDIRS Midwifery Digest* 9 (3): 327–30.

Smith, N. (1999a) Men in antenatal classes teaching 'the whole birth thing'. *Practising Midwife* 2 (1): 23–6.

Smith, N.J. (1999c) Antenatal classes and the transition to fatherhood: a study of some fathers' views. *MIDIRS Midwifery Digest* 9 (4): 463–8.

Smith, R. (2000) Babies and consent: yet another NHS scandal. *British Medical Journal* 320 (7245): 1285–6.

Somers-Smith, M.J. (1999) A place for the partner? Expectations and experiences of support during childbirth. *Midwifery* 15 (2): 101–8.

Speak, M. and Aitken-Swan, J. (1982) *Male Midwives – A Report of Two Studies.* London: DHSS.

Spock, B. (1979) *Baby and Child Care* (4th edn). London: The Bodley Head.

Stanko, E.A. (1997) Models of understanding violence against women (ch. 2, p. 13), in S. Bewley, J. Friend and G. Mezey (eds) *Violence Against Women*. London: RCOG Press.

Stanway, A. (1984) *Infertility: A Common-sense Guide for the Childless* (2nd edn). Wellingborough: Thorsons.

Stark, E., Flitcraft, A., Zuckerman, D., Grey, A., Robison, J. and Frazier, W. (1981) Wife abuse in the medical setting. *Domestic Violence Monograph Series* 7: 7–41.

Steinberg, S., Kruckman, L. and Steinberg, S. (2000) Reinventing fatherhood in Japan and Canada. *Social Science and Medicine* 50: 1257–72.

Stephens, L. (1998) Male power: a challenge to normal childbirth. *British Journal of Midwifery* 6 (7): 450–3.

Sternas, K.A., O'Hare, P., Lehman, K. and Milligan, R. (1999) Nursing and medical student teaming for service learning in partnership with the community: an emerging holistic model for interdisciplinary education and practice. *Holistic Nursing Practice* 13 (2): 66–77.

Storr, G.B. (2003) *It Takes Three to Breastfeed: Uncovering the Role of the Father.* Unpublished Ph.D. thesis, University of Edinburgh, p. 52.

Stroebe, M. and Schut, H. (1995) The dual process model of coping with bereavement: rationale and description. *Death Studies* 23 (3): 197–224.

Stroebe, W. and Stroebe, M.S. (1987) *Bereavement and Health: The Psychological and Physical Consequences of Partner Loss.* Cambridge: Cambridge University Press.

Sullivan-Lyons, J. (1998) Men becoming fathers: 'Sometimes I wonder how I'll cope' (ch. 12, pp. 227–44), in S. Clement (ed.) *Psychological Perspectives on Pregnancy and Childbirth*. Edinburgh: Churchill Livingstone.

Summersgill, P. (1993) Couvade – the retaliation of marginalised fathers (ch. 6, pp. 91–109), in J. Alexander, V. Levy and S. Roch (eds) *Midwifery Practice: A Research-based Approach*. London: Macmillan.

Tamimi, R.M., Lagiou, P., Mucci, L.A., Hsieh, C.C., Adami, H.O. and Trichopoulos, D. (2003) Average energy intake among pregnant women carrying a boy compared with a girl. *British Medical Journal* 7326(7401): 1245–6.

Tew, M. (1984) Planned and unplanned deliveries at home. *British Medical Journal* 288 (6431): 1691–2.

Tew, M. (1995) *Safer Childbirth? A Critical History of Maternity Care* (2nd edn). London: Chapman and Hall.

Thacker, S.B., Stroup, D. and Chang, M. (2002) Continuous electronic heart rate monitoring for fetal assessment during labor (Cochrane Review), in *The Cochrane Library*, Issue 1. Oxford: Update Software.

Thomas, P. (2002) The midwife you have called knows you are waiting. . . . A consumer view (ch. 2, pp. 20–38), in R. Mander and V. Fleming (eds) *Failure to Progress: The Contraction of the Midwifery Profession*. London: Routledge.

Thomas, S.G. and Upton, D. (2000) Expectant fathers' attitudes towards pregnancy. *British Journal of Midwifery* 8 (4): 218–21.

Thompson, N. (1997) Masculinity and loss (ch. 4, p. 76), in D. Field, J. Hockey and N. Small (eds) *Death, Gender and Ethnicity*. London: Routledge.

Thomson, A. (1989) Why don't women breast feed? (ch. 11, p. 215), in S. Robinson and A. Thomson (ed.) *Midwives Research and Childbirth*, Vol. 1. London: Chapman and Hall.

Tosh, J. (1999) *A Man's Place: Masculinity and the Middle-Class Home in Victorian England*. New Haven, CT: Yale University Press.

Tosh, J. (2000) *The Pursuit of History* (3rd edn). Harlow: Pearson Education.

Towler, J. and Bramall, J. (1986) *Midwives in History and Society*. London: Croom Helm.

Townsend, N. (1999) Fatherhoods and fieldwork: intersections between personal and theoretical positions. *Men and Masculinities* 2 (1): 87–97.

Trethowan, W.H. and Conlon, M.F. (1965) The Couvade Syndrome. *British Journal of Psychiatry* 111, 57–66.

TVS (2002) The pregnancy scanner. Technology Ventures Scotland. http://www.technologyscotland.org/pioneering/body_pregnancy.html. Accessed 18 February.

Tylor, E.B. (1865) *Researches into the Early History of Mankind and the Development of Civilisation*. London: John Murray.

UKCC (2001) Supporting women who intend to give birth at home. Registrar's letter 21/2001, 31 August. http://www.ukcc.org.uk/cms/content/home/search.asp.

Ursano, R.J. and McCarroll, J.E. (1995) Exposure to traumatic death: the nature of the stressor (ch. 3), in R.J. Ursano, B.G. McCaughey and C.S. Fullerton (eds) *Individual and Community Responses to Trauma and Disaster*. Cambridge: Cambridge University Press.

Van Gennep, A. (1960) The rites of passage. Translated by M.B. Vizedom and G.L. Caffee. London: Routledge & Kegan Paul.

Vance, J.C., Boyle, F.M., Najman, J.M. and Thearle, M.J. (2002) Couple distress after sudden infant or perinatal death: A 30 month follow up. *Journal of Paediatrics and Child Health* 38: 368–72.

Varney Burst, H. (1983) The influence of consumers in the birthing movement. *Topics in Clinical Nursing* 5: 42–54.

Vehvilainen-Julkunen, K. (1995) Family training: supporting mothers and fathers in the transition to parenthood. *Journal of Advanced Nursing* 22 (4): 731–7.

Vehvilainen-Julkunen, K. and Liukkonen, A. (1998) Fathers' experiences of childbirth. *Midwifery* 14 (1): 10–17.

Viisainen, K. (2001) Negotiating control and meaning: home birth as a self-constructed choice in Finland. *Social Science and Medicine* 52 (7): 1109–21.

Vincent-Priya, J. (1992) *Birth Traditions and Modern Pregnancy Care*. Shaftesbury: Element.

Wagner, M. (1994) *Pursuing the Birth Machine: The Search for Appropriate Birth Technology*. Camperdown: Ace Graphics.

Wahlstrom, O., Sanden, I. and Hammar, M. (1997) Multiprofessional education in the medical curriculum. *Medical Education* 31 (6): 425–9.

Walker, J., McCarthy, P. and Simpson, B. (2002) Renegotiating fatherhood. Newcastle Centre for Family Studies. http://www.ncl.ac.uk/ncfs/ncfs/document32.html. Accessed 20 May.

Walker, J.F. (1976) Midwife or obstetric nurse? Some perceptions of midwives and obstetricians of the role of the midwife. *Journal of Advanced Nursing* 1: 129–38.

Walker, L. (1979) *The Battered Woman*. New York: Harper & Row.

Wallace, E.M., MacKintosh, C.L., Brownlee, M., Laidlaw, L. and Johnstone, F.D. (1995) An observational study of midwife–medical staff interaction in a labour ward environment. *Journal of Obstetrics and Gynaecology* 15 (3): 165–70.

Wallach, H. (1982) *Psychological and Physiological Childbirth-related Variables Affecting Pain of Labour*. Unpublished Master's thesis, Lakehead University.

Walsh, D. (2000a) Evidence-based care. Part three: Assessing women's progress in labour. *British Journal of Midwifery* 8 (7): 449–57.

Walsh, D. (2000b) Evidence-based care. Part four: Fetal monitoring should be controlled. *British Journal of Midwifery* 8 (8): 511–16.

Ward, S. and Spence, A. (2002) Training midwives to screen for domestic violence. *MIDIRS Midwifery Digest* Supplement 1: S15–17.

Waterman, A.S. (1999) Identity, the identity statuses, and identity status development: a contemporary statement. *Developmental Review* 19 (4): 591–621.

Watson, N. and Mander, R. (1995) Advertising infant formula in the maternity area. *MIDIRS Midwifery Digest* 5 (3): 338–41.

Weaver, J. (2002) Court-ordered caesarean sections (ch. 13, pp. 229–48), in A. Bainham, S.D. Sclater and M. Richards (eds) *Body Lore and Laws: Essays on Law and the Human Body*. Oxford: Hart.

Wenger, G.C. and Burholt, V. (2001) Differences over time in older people's relationships with children, grandchildren, nieces and nephews in rural North Wales. *Ageing and Society* 21: 567–90.

Whelan, A. and Lupton, P. (1998) Promoting successful breast feeding among women with a low income. *Midwifery* 14 (2): 94–100.

Wickham, S. (2000) Evidence informed midwifery. *MIDIRS Midwifery Digest* 10 (2): 149–50.

Williams, J. (1997) The controlling power of childbirth in Britain (ch. 11, p. 232), in H. Marland and A.M. Rafferty (eds) *Midwives, Society and Childbirth*. London: Routledge.

Willocks, J. (1986) Scottish man-midwives in 18th century London (ch. 4, p. 45), in D.A. Dow (ed.) *The Influence of Scottish Medicine*. Carnforth: Parthenon.

Willocks, J. (1996) Medical ultrasound: a Glasgow development which swept the World University of Glasgow. *Avenue No. 19*: January. http://www.gla.ac.uk/Graduate/Avenue/19/5medical.htm. Accessed 18 February 2002.

Wilson, A (1995) *The Making of Man-Midwifery*. London: UCL Press.

Wilson, A.C., Forsyth, J.S., Greene, S.A., Irvine, L., Hau, C. and Howie, P.W. (1998) Relation of infant diet to childhood health: seven year follow up of cohort of children in Dundee infant feeding study. *British Medical Journal* 316 (7124): 21–5.

Witz, A. (1992) Medical men and midwives (ch. 4, pp. 104–27), in A. Witz *Professions and Patriarchy*. London: Routledge.

Women's Aid (2001) About women's aid. National Federation of Women's Aid. http://www.womensaid.org.uk/about/index.htm. Accessed 14 August 2002.

Woollett, A. and Dosanjh-Matwala, N. (1990) Postnatal care: the attitudes and experiences of Asian women in East London. *Midwifery* 6 (4): 178–84.

Woollett, A. and Parr, M. (1997) Psychological tasks for women and men in the postpartum. *Journal of Reproductive and Infant Psychology* 15 (2): 159–83.

Woollett, A., White, D. and Lyon, L. (1982) Observation of fathers at birth (ch. 4, pp. 72–93), in N. Beail and J. McGuire (eds) *Fathers: Psychological Perspectives*. London: Junction Books.

Zain, H.A., Wright. J.W., Parrish, G.E. and Diehl, S.J. (1998) Interpreting the fetal heart rate tracing. Effect of knowledge of neonatal outcome. *Journal of Reproductive Medicine* 43 (4): 367–70.

Index